Don't Get Thin Get Healthy

by Loraine Holden, MS

to Stan & Carole

for good health

Loraine Holden

Published by Golden Green Press

Fair Oaks, California

Library of Congress Cataloging-In-Publication Data:

Holden, Loraine

    Don't Get thin Get Healthy / Loraine Holden

    Includes bibliographical reference and index

    ISBN 0-9755064-0-4

    1. Health 2. Aging 3. Exercise 4. Nutrition

    Library of Congress Control Number: 2005921856

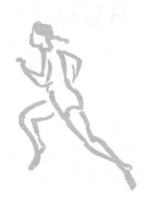

ISBN 0-9755064-0-4

Illustrations ©2005, Warren L. Dayton

Published by Golden Green Press

PO Box 1087 • Fair Oaks, CA 95628-1087

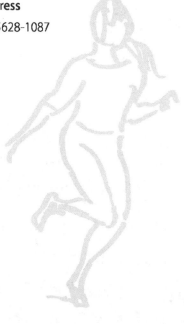

About The Author

"I'm not just a scientist who gives cold facts from books and research. I would like the reader to think of me like an elder who can impart wisdom gained during a long, eventful life." --Loraine Holden

Loraine Holden has a broad background in biology and medicine. Her experience combines hands-on work with patients and studying the relationships of biochemistry and disease. Her M.S. degree dealt with the cytochrome enzymes.

She attended medical school at the University of Colorado for more than three years, and conducted research at the University of Rochester, Hahnemann University and the University of Colorado in biochemistry and physiology. She did library research and technical writing for Smith Kline and French Pharmaceutical Co. She has taught college courses in anatomy, physiology and bacteriology.

Loraine is an ardent advocate for exercise. She feels that learning physical skills produces confidence and reduces stress. She has overcome arthritis and other ailments and wants to help others gain a long and vigorous life.

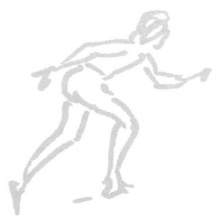

Acknowledgments

I did not try to cite the many authors and sources I had consulted to write this book. Special thanks go to doctors Michael R. Eades and Mary Dan Eades for their permission to use the cholesterol chart from Protein Power Life Plan, and a description of one of their patients from Protein Power who looks like four different people, depending on his lifestyle. Janeen Hunt let me use her annotated bibliography on fat and cholesterol to give credence to a viewpoint at odds with popular thought. The Oldways Preservation Trust allowed me to reproduce their four healthy food pyramids.

In numerous anecdotes, when possible I asked for permission to use them. Sometimes I changed the names and details. If any persons think they recognize themselves, I extend my thanks. They can appreciate the fact they are helping other people with similar problems. I thank those at an anti-aging seminar at Steiner College in Fair Oaks who filled out my questionnaire. I didn't use their information but it helped launch this book.

I want to thank Ruth Younger for manuscript suggestions, Libbie Martin for major editing and Mary Alice Coverdale for final editing. Also Anita Thomas and Martha Dayton of Binding Plus (www.bindingplus.com) for publishing services and book design, and Warren L. Dayton at ArtiFact, Ink (design@printsofpeace.com) for illustrations.

Disclaimer

Contents

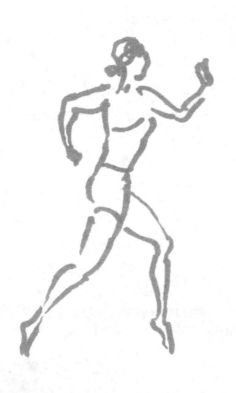

The Golden Mean...

Are you one of the millions of people tired of a diet "quick fix" that works in the short term but can't be followed year in and year out? You don't want to be among the 90 percent of dieters who gain back all the fat they lost and later suffer a debilitating old age. You want something that lets you live a normal life and stay fit and healthy. You don't know what to try next.

Let me guide you through the underbrush of conflicting claims in the scores of health books on the market. You can have a healthy body and keep it the rest of your life. Here's how:

Avoid Extremes

Aristotle, the ancient Greek philosopher (384-322 BC) had the right idea for a good life. He said to aim for the "Golden Mean." A mean is like an average. It's what Goldilocks discovered when she tasted Baby Bear's porridge. It was neither too hot nor too cold – it was just right. Strive for a Golden Mean in all aspects of health, a middle area with room for individual differences. Your body physiology can be as unique as your appearance.

Like you, I have gone on extreme diets and got very thin, then regained those pounds plus many more. When I stopped dieting and concentrated on my health, I have kept my weight within four pounds of 120 for more than 30 years. I'm well over 60 and have abundant energy. I eat healthful foods, use very few supplements or prescriptions and get plenty of exercise.

I can help you get similar results, whatever your age. If you're in your teens or twenties you might be lucky and feel invulnerable. Nothing seems to happen no matter what you eat or how little you exercise. You'll find out later that bad habits can later produce minor aches and pains, then major health problems. Some of you are in your thirties and noticing the first signs of aging. Many are in your fifties starting to think about retirement. Others are in your senior years suffering from medical maladies and broken bones and going to the funerals of your friends.

It is predicted that 25 percent of Americans who reach the age of 70 will live to be 100. Other studies show that a third of people age 85 or older get Alzheimer's Disease. But these statistics don't have to apply to you. You can be among those who stay healthy.

Many of you are concerned about losing body fat, so the first section of the book will analyze various diets, their rationales and the effects on body chemistry. Some programs are based on misinformation.

In assessing diets and their benefits, I ask the following questions: Can you get all the nutrients necessary for health by eating raw foods or abstaining from meat and other animal products? Do you need specific combinations of foods or certain ratios of carbohydrate, protein and fat? Must you supplement any diet with extra vitamins and many micro-nutrients? Though we're all human, there are slight differences in our cellular enzymes as well as our external appearance.

There is a Golden Mean

What you consume rarely has to be all or nothing. There is a Golden Mean. I'll point out the advantages of some of the diets and valid points made by various authors. You can decide the best program for your body type and your schedule. You can vary it with your activities. A candy bar can turn to fat if you're sitting around, but it can give you added energy during vigorous hiking.

No magic pill can substitute for healthful foods. With good basic health and a minimum number of vitamins or other supplements, you won't need a lot of medications. Many seniors take 10 to 20 different prescriptions, any one of which can interfere with the others or cause side effects. Moreover, most drugs control symptoms but don't eliminate the basic causes of disease.

Neither is there a silver bullet that can vanquish all the problems of aging, but exercise comes the closest to being a "miracle." Vigorous exercises can stimulate your body to produce age-defying chemicals to prevent debilitating symptoms as you get older. You need various forms of exercise to help your heart and lungs, your bones and muscles and your brain. *Any* exercise is better than *no exercise.* The best is the one you do consistently, even if it doesn't have all the components. It's even better if the exercise is fun and done with other people. As your body gets healthier, you will be able to increase the duration and vary the types of exercise.

Your mental attitude can help maintain optimum health

Finally, good attitude helps you deal with stress and counteracts stress hormones. A positive or spiritual outlook can often help as well. Even if certain authors use faulty reasoning in advocating their diets, their up-beat or spiritual emphasis makes up for this. The mind-body connection is very real. Love of a friend or a pet can help keep you healthy.

Besides diet, exercise and mental attitude, you also need to avoid harmful chemicals in your food and in your environment.

The cost of medical care is increasing tremendously every year. Hospital costs are spiraling out of reach and more people are unable to afford health insurance. It costs more to neglect your body than to stay well. Despite medical advances, more people are suffering from metabolic maladies like diabetes and heart disease. Symptoms are treated, but the diseases are not cured. Who is going to pay to treat the chronic conditions of an aging population? Is it logical to assume that Medicare or an insurance company can always pay for the latest life saving methods or apparatus?

What kind of life will you have in your later years?

Will you be healthy enough to remain in your own home? Will you end up in a nursing home? Cancer and heart disease are still the big killers of people over 50. Many of you will survive a stroke or heart attack. You may have your cancer treated all right, but at a cost in time, money and suffering. Even though medical science has made great advances in organ transplants and chemotherapy, wouldn't it be better not to endure these expensive, unpleasant procedures? You can improve your health, your appearance, your energy and your outlook for your full life span.

Your quality of life now and in your later years depends on your taking care of your health. It is better to avoid debilitating illness and live a full life in a healthy body. It is never too late to start.

Your body is meant to be healthy. You just have to give it the means. This book will provide the means to a fit, healthy body, avoiding debilitating aging. Keep in mind, your goal is not getting thin but getting healthy.

Start by asking yourself the following questions:

1   Are you dissatisfied with the way your body looks? If yes, is it because you don't look like celebrities on television or the movies? Read the chapters on Fat Phobia and Measuring What Is Normal, Too Thin or Obese.

2   Do you accept as truth statements from hearsay, the radio, television or magazines? Read Myths and Misinformation, as well as the many chapters on Body Chemistry. Even doctors and other scientists can interpret data according to a personal bias. What is true for animals or a select group of people like marathon runners might not apply to you.

3   Do you want instant gratification – a quick-fix with a pill or extreme diet? Wouldn't you rather have a change that lasts the rest of your life?

4   Do you expect a prescription every time you see a doctor? Advertisements tell you to ask for the latest drugs. Doctors oblige, having received brochures and free samples from representatives of pharmaceutical companies.

5   Do you measure the value of everything in terms of its cost? Do you think a generic drug can't be as good as one that costs much more?

6 Are you willing to pay higher taxes now or in the future that increase the profits of drug companies? Most drugs only alleviate symptoms, but don't cure or even prevent disease.

7 Do you go along with "experts" who, at the stroke of a pen, transform the values of your previously normal blood chemistry into something that requires expensive medication?

8 When you're retired, will you be willing to buy drugs that cost more than your monthly food budget? Or do you expect someone else to pick up the tab?

9 Which would you rather do – have surgery to clean out or replace diseased arteries or prevent the conditions that cause them? Does a repeat operation make sense to you? Wouldn't you rather change your habits to give your body the chance to repair itself so you won't need surgery or a lot of medications?

10 Do you want to get healthy and stay healthy so you can remain in your own home without fear of debilitating accidents? Would you be willing to change your lifestyle? Will you try diets and exercises that slowly repair your faulty metabolism and give you a firm, fit body?

You can aim for the Golden Mean of ageless, good health.

You have the power to choose!

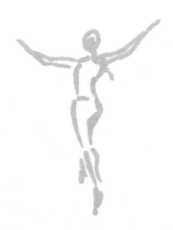

Body Image & Fat Phobia

"Help! I need to find a bathing suit that doesn't make me look fat."

The comic strip character Cathy, penned by Cathy Guisewaite, echoes the cries of women in fitting rooms everywhere.

In the last 15 years, the fashion trend in bathing suits has resulted in suits cut to reveal more and more hip. This change has left most otherwise "normal" women dissatisfied.

It used to be that the length of the leg was not emphasized, except for the leotards of ballet dancers. They wore tights underneath so no skin was revealed. That same high cut on a bathing suit shows the average woman that she has fat on her buttocks. She doesn't look like the athletes in the Olympics or what is shown as the ideal body in advertisements, television or movies.

Manufacturers make more money when women are dissatisfied with how they look. When women can't look like models in the media, self-esteem plummets and they usually go to one of two extremes: either they starve themselves or comfort themselves with unhealthy food.

What can today's woman do?

Several years ago she had choices. Many bathing suits had skirts. Others minimized real or imagined figure flaws. Since she can't find a bathing suit that covers more of her anatomy, a woman can only try to change her body to fit the suit. This can have a negative effect on her health.

Dr. Christiane Northrup in *Women's Bodies, Women's Wisdom*

says that while a gymnast may have less than 18 percent body fat, a normal healthy woman has between 22 percent and 28 percent. Women with enough estrogen are supposed to have a certain amount of fat, including fat on the buttocks. According to Dr. Northrup, a woman is anorexic at 10 percent fat, which makes it impossible for her body to produce enough female hormones. As women and girls try to fit an impossible stereotype, anorexia and bulimia are increasing dramatically. Meanwhile, the use of diet products, exercise machines, fitness clubs and personal trainers has skyrocketed.

Your height and musculature affect the amount of food you can eat and not get fat

A tall woman whose skin presents a greater surface area for heat loss needs more calories. She can eat more without putting on fat than a short woman of the same weight. Similarly, someone who builds more muscle by exercise can have bigger meals and not get fat.

The average woman must work with what she has. In the animal world, a gazelle is lithe and slim. The zebra, another grazing animal, has a firm rounded body. Billions of dollars are spent on products and services that make every woman think she should look like a gazelle. In most cases, failure is inevitable. The woman who doesn't want the curves of a zebra can end up looking like a hippo when she slows down her metabolism with crash diets. As her body hangs on to every calorie she takes in, she ends up with more pounds that are harder to lose after each diet

As a teenager, I thought 123 pounds was too much for someone 5'3" tall. Since I didn't like the fatter thighs that came with puberty, I walked five to seven miles a day and dieted with intensity. For two years, I consumed only vegetables, lean meat and non-fat milk. Then desiring grains and fruits, I counted carbohydrates as well as total calories. I yo-yoed between 102 and 137 pounds for many years, feeling guilty if I ever succumbed to any sweets. Like an alcoholic who fell off the wagon, I would then eat many portions of candy or a rich sweet dessert. Since I always vowed to give them up the rest of my life I wanted to enjoy a last fling.

Then I talked to a former stewardess who said she had kept her weight within the limits imposed by the airline by putting her finger down her throat to induce vomiting. I felt even more unworthy and guilty when I tried that method to undo the eating of forbidden foods.

After accepting that I will always have some fat on my short thighs, I stopped dieting. My weight has varied between 116 and 124 pounds for years on a nutritious, well-balanced diet that includes fats. I eat an occasional dessert without guilt or weight gain. I don't look like a movie star but I'm a healthy example of my body type. With my short thighs I will never be like a gazelle.

Fat has become like a dirty word

Fat is something to be avoided both on your plate and on your body. People are desperate to try anything that promises fat loss. Manufacturers make more money if you are dissatisfied with your body. Advertisers then sell low-fat or no-fat foods. Delicious looking bran muffins are labeled "low fat," but the first, most plentiful ingredient is sugar. Consumers don't know that the body easily turns sugars into fat. Now the craze for "low-carb." foods has caused the production of high-protein bars. Protein can also be changed into fat, especially if you're sedentary.

Fat hasn't always had a bad name. In prehistoric times, images of fat earth goddesses were revered as symbols of abundance. In later centuries, fat meant both fertility and survival in many cultures. A fat woman would be able to conceive and nurse her babies even in periods when food was scarce. Reuben's nudes from Renaissance times were ample women. Such women could better withstand diseases like tuberculosis. In the nineteenth and twentieth centuries, thin women like Mimi in the opera *La Boheme* had pretty faces but died young from that wasting disease. The ability to put on body fat is built into the genes for survival of the human race.

Current fashion produces a changing popular body type

When survival wasn't an issue, women tried to change their bodies to conform to what culture defined as beautiful. In East Asia, girls had metal rings put around their necks to make them longer. Little Chinese girls had their feet folded and tightly bound with strips of cloth to make them tiny. A century ago, European and American women wore tight corsets to get a wasp waist. In the 1920s, as women wore shorter skirts, the ideal body type was that of a young adolescent.

In the 1940s and 1950s, the ideal woman in the movies had enough body fat to give her typical feminine curves, but with a trim waistline. Films showed a range of beautiful body types from Audrey Hepburn to Marilyn Monroe. Some were even short. Average women got brainwashed when they saw the ultra-thin British model, Twiggy, in the movie *The Boy Friend* and the lithe young body of Brooke Shields in *Blue Lagoon*. About then I remember seeing a new billboard for suntan lotion. The shapely bathing beauty had been replaced by one who had long thin thighs.

Models became even thinner to show off the clothes they were displaying and others wanted the same look. Accepting the adage that "You can't be too thin or too rich," upper-class women tried to look like emaciated models. Formerly beautiful healthy debutantes bragged about dieting down to less than 100 pounds. In Tom Wolfe's book, *Bonfire of the Vanities*, the men in their social circles called such women *x-rays* because they had so little flesh on their bones. On Mary Tyler Moore's television show, her friend Rhoda was always dieting, even though she never looked overweight. Later, her picture in a tabloid newspaper showed her as a gaunt, thin woman, proud of shedding the pounds she didn't need to lose.

More women of normal weight thought they should lose 10 or 15 pounds. The sales of diet products increased. Many diets produced a temporary weight loss and then slowed down the dieters' metabolism. Most people gained back the lost weight and added more. The extreme diets had made them first lose muscle and then start losing fat. The later weight gain was mostly fat. When a person tried the next low-calorie diet, it was harder to lose the fat. Now, more than half of the adult population has become obese because of dieting and our sedentary lifestyle.

Many women stick with a low-calorie diet and control their appetite by smoking

Some indeed stay thin. However, smoking is a much greater health risk than obesity. The members' magazine of the Kaiser Permanente health plan says you would have to be 100 or more pounds overweight to be as unhealthy as a smoker. A thin friend of mine in San Diego was admired because of her nice figure at age 50. Two years later she died of lung cancer from tobacco smoke. Who wants to be a beautiful corpse?

Yet girls and young women are so anxious to be thin they ignore the consequences of using cigarettes. An article in the November 2000 *Popular Science* shows a steady increase in smoking. In 1991, 27.5 percent of teens smoked. By 1999, it was 34.8 percent. Many college women are vegetarians and exercise for health, but disregard the long-term effects of cigarettes.

We are still trying to change our basic anatomy even in our modern civilized society

We might be affluent enough to show we don't need to store body fat for a possible period of famine. But are we really civilized if we reject a healthy natural body type and glorify emaciated bodies similar to those of concentration camp survivors? If average women weren't bombarded with images of very thin women, they could just exercise more and eat a wide variety of unprocessed foods to keep from getting fat. Better to be a healthy Venus de Milo than try to be thin and end up obese. Fat is not the enemy. The real enemies are a culture that dictates a specific body shape and multibillion-dollar industries that profit when people try to conform to an unrealistic image.

What You Can Do

- Watch some movies made in the 1950s and notice the more shapely actresses.

- Check with the men in your life. Do they prefer a rounded bottom or a flat one?

- Look honestly at your own particular dimensions and frame. Just as all animals don't look like gazelles, all humans shouldn't try for an impossible look dictated by advertisers or the media.

- Don't try to lose fat with unhealthy crash diets that always have a rebound effect.

- Don't try to control your weight by smoking.

- Rebel against those businesses that promote a particular body image and make you dissatisfied with your body to keep their profits rolling in.

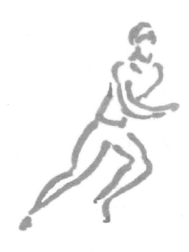

What is Normal, Too Thin or Obese?

Experts in diet, exercise and health disagree on what should be a normal weight.

The average American is getting fatter while trying to look like the ideal shown in the media. According to Dr. Christiane Northrup, the average Miss America weighed *134 pounds in 1954* and 117 pounds in 1980. The decline has continued. The average fashion model weighed 8 percent less than a normal young woman in the 1970s. By 1998, the typical model weighed 25 percent less — an impossible goal for the average girl without endangering her health. Even a female runner shouldn't get below 18 percent fat or she will stop menstruating and have thinner, weaker bones despite the positive aspects of exercise.

The media perpetuates an ultra-thin myth that is NOT healthy for most people. Nobody wants to be fat, but do they really want to be thin? What's wrong with a healthy medium?

Weight is only one indicator to determine if we need to reduce

The old insurance charts derived from weights that include clothing and shoes are useless. A recent United States Department of Agriculture (USDA) chart doesn't help either. It has weights for a person over 35 of either sex that range from 108 to 138 pounds for someone 5 feet tall. For a person 5' 6", it was 130 to 167 lbs. and for someone 6 feet tall, 155 to 199 lbs. I assume women should be at the lower weights and men at the higher. But men and women don't have the same physiological make-up. They should have different charts reflecting those differences. A simple rule of thumb from 50 years ago was that anyone 5 feet tall should weigh 100 pounds. A woman would add another 5 pounds for each additional inch. Men, with their higher proportion of muscle and heavier bones, would add 7 pounds for each additional inch.

Approximations can vary with body type

Teen-age girls are taller and narrower today. One man can have muscles and well-distributed fat but another of the same height and weight can have a fat belly and thin arms and legs, similar to many cadavers in my Medical Anatomy class. The exception was a man in his thirties who had died in an auto accident. He was well-built, with a quarter-inch of fat over all his muscles just under the skin.

The charts don't always reflect reality. For example, according to standard charts a heavy athlete would be obese even though his extra weight is muscle. His body build is different from that of a runner. They should not be judged by the same standard. In *Gary Null's Ultimate Anti-Aging Program*, Null says the leaner you are, the healthier. Runner Gary Null suggests a rule of thumb of 106 lbs. for a man standing 5 feet tall and 6 pounds more for each added inch. He doesn't consider that a muscular weight lifter may have 8 to 10 pounds for each inch over five feet.

Calculate your Body Mass Index (BMI) to see if you're too thin, normal, or overweight

Robert Haas says BMI = weight in pounds times 703 divided by the height in inches squared. (Other authors multiply by 705 instead of 703). Haas says the normal BMI should be between 19 and 22. For example a 5'3" woman would multiply her 120 lbs. by 703 to get 84360. Divide this by 63 x 63 [3869] and get a BMI of 21.8.) The formula wouldn't work for pregnant or nursing women.

Body builders or sedentary elderly are other exceptions. A male acquaintance, age 86, weighs 165 pounds and is 5'8" tall. His BMI is 165 x 703 = 115995, divided by 68 x 68 equals 25, a high BMI. This older man looks medium to thin. Having retained muscle mass over the years, he would be another exception to any standard BMI value. He is not overweight.

You won't need to calculate your BMI if you use one of the

many Body Mass Index charts on the Internet. These give a general average. Most charts say a BMI of 20-22 is ideal, 22-25 is still healthy, 25-30 is overweight, and more than 30 is obese.

Obesity should be defined as having an unhealthy amount of fat

More people do have excess fat now than 30 years ago, but are more than 50 percent of Americans obese? Many books now say if you weigh more than 20 percent over the norm, you are obese. They reflect the most recent guidelines from the National Institutes of Health, which, with the stroke of a pen, classified 29 million more adults as obese. In other words, if a 5'4" woman should weigh 120 pounds, she would be *obese* at 144!

Back in the 1950s, a Hollywood critic said the Italian movie actress in the film *Bitter Rice* was 30 pounds overweight and would never succeed in the U.S. I saw her in that one movie. She wasn't obese, just a trim healthy-looking medium. Judy Garland might still be alive if movie moguls hadn't insisted she get thin and stay thin. Her daughter, Liza Minelli, has resisted that pressure. Better to be alive with a few extra pounds than dead.

Percentage of body fat is not the same as BMI - it can be measured in various ways

These methods give only an approximation and results can differ depending on the method used. The graph accompanying the chapter summarizes the recommended body fat from various sources. Some consider only the active adult and don't mention those over 60. Kaiser has an average within age groups instead of giving a range of healthy percentages of fat. Recommendations were that a woman's maximum fat from ages 19-24 should be 21.9 percent; at 25-29 years, 22.4 percent; at 30-34 years, 22.7 percent; at 35-39 years, 23.7 percent; at 40-44 years, 25.4 percent; at 45-49 years, 27.2 percent; and at 50-59 years, 30 percent. At more than 60 years, it should not be more than 30.8 percent. I stepped on the scales at Kaiser, then used the electronic grips and punched in the criteria of age, height, whether athletic and if clothed. Heavy winter clothing and shoes probably made a difference. My total body fat was said to be 27.9 percent.

I put my heel into an apparatus provided by Sutter Davis Hospital at a health fair. Using age, height and the weight on their scale, fat mass was determined by the BIA (Bio-Electric Impedance Analysis) method. My body fat was 29 percent, but their sheet said results might not be accurate because of exercise within 12 hours or consuming food, water, alcohol, caffeine or diuretics within four hours. See the Ideal Body Fat table for a comparison with other methods.

In the book, *Protein Power*, Dr. Michael Eades and Dr. Mary Dan Eades have complicated charts to determine body fat. A woman measures her waist, hips and height, all in inches. Hip and waist measurements are converted to other numbers and subtracted from another factor related to height to get percentage of body fat. With this method, I have about 26 percent body fat.

A man's wrist circumference is subtracted from waist measurement to account for bone structure. Where this number intersects with his weight on another chart indicates a man's percentage of body fat. The Eades don't describe the source of the factors used but their methods roughly correlate with other ways of determining fat, as shown in the tables later in the chapter.

You can determine body fat by pinching the skin

You may have heard the saying, "If you can pinch an inch, that part of your body is too fat." Cliff Sheats in *Lean Bodies Total Fitness* says to determine your body fat by having an expert use calipers to pinch skin folds on five different parts of your body:

1. Triceps. [This muscle hangs down from the upper arm and jiggles unless you're very fit. One 70-year-old thin friend says she has enough excess tissue there to make another arm.]
2. Abdominal vertical fold an inch to one side and one inch below the navel
3. Iliac crest, just over the hip bone
4. Sub-scapular area, an inch from the bottom of the shoulder blade toward the spine
5. Front of the thigh, half way between the knee and hip.

Forget all the measurements and Sheats' complicated formula.

Just see if you can pinch more than one inch of flab around the abdomen and in other places you can reach.

Covert Bailey, in *New Fit or Fat,* says he uses skin fold measurements in his clinic because they're convenient. He says body fat can be overestimated in a fit person but in a flabby one might be underestimated because it doesn't measure internal abdominal fat. Bailey says a method with the total body under water is more accurate. It never understates body fat but can give too high a reading if the person doesn't exhale completely or has gas in the intestine.

Body fat percentage ideals for men and women

Ideal Percentage of Body Fat in Women according to various sources:

Source	to age 40	to age 60	after age 60
Sutter Health	21 % to 30 %	24 % to 34 %	25% to 35 %
Eades		21 % to 27 %	22 % to 31 %
Northrup		20% to 28%	
Bailey	22 % to 23 %		
Sheats	19 % to 24 %		
Kaiser (modified)	21.9% to 23.7%	25.4 % to 30%	Less than 30.8%

Ideal Percentage of Body Fat in Men according to various sources:

Source	to age 40	to age 60	after age 60
Sutter Health	9 % to 20 %	12 % to 22 %	14 % to 25 %
Eades		13 % to 19 %	17 % to 21 %
Bailey	15 %		
Sheats	13 % to 16 %		
Null	7 % to 10 %		

You can use a simple method in a swimming pool to see if your percentage of body fat is in a healthy range. Bailey says to float on your back with full lungs. Blow out all your air and see if you start sinking. A person with more than 25 percent fat still floats easily. A woman with a healthy 22-23 percent can float with shallow breaths. A man with a healthy 15 percent of fat sinks. At below 13 percent fat, even with full lungs, he sinks. [As taught in a life-saving class, body position can make a difference. Some men who think they can't float can hang vertically in the water if the arms are stretched out forward on the surface.]

Both Sheats and Bailey say to forget using the scales, but every two to six months check on body fat using calipers on skin folds. Some authors are extreme, suggesting a man should have 7-10 percent body fat and a woman about 12-14 percent body fat. I say a woman with that little body fat is eating too little and exercising too much. She is dangerously anorexic. It's irresponsible to say a woman should be so thin. Too much anorexia and bulimia exist already, even among pre-teens.

Distribution of fat is the most important factor in correlating obesity with certain diseases

Medical professionals say a pear-shaped woman, with most of her fat in her hips and thighs, is healthier than one of similar weight whose abdominal fat gives her an apple shape. The excess fat in men is almost always around the waist. Fat deposited under the skin is not nearly as dangerous as that around the vital organs in the abdominal cavity.

Internal abdominal fat correlates with heart disease as well as diabetes and other degenerative diseases. In other words, soft fat just under the skin over the abdominal muscles is much less dangerous than fat under the muscle layer and around the internal organs. Certain internal fat, like that around the kidneys, is never lost. A piece of tissue called the omentum, shaped like an apron draped over the intestines, can collect a lot of fat in the sedentary overeater. If you can pinch more than an inch of the soft fat on your belly, it is unsightly. If your abdomen is solid but round, that can be a great deal less healthy.

One of my tennis partners had such a fat distribution, having developed strong abdominal muscles in skiing and other sports. Most of his fat was around his internal organs. He had a good tailor and looked the typical rotund 50 year old professional man. Once, when we went to a popular restaurant with a long line, he gave his last name prefaced with "Doctor" and asked the hostess, "Can we get a table right away? I might need to go to the hospital to deliver a baby." She took a look at his portly belly and said sweetly, "Oh my, you do look far along, but our policy is to seat patrons in the order they arrive." If a man looks pregnant, he has dangerous internal fat.

The stomach can be permanently stretched. One cat dissected in my introductory anatomy class was a large tom with excess fat in his abdominal cavity. Instead of a contracted stomach like normal cats, this cat's stomach had permanently stretched. If a human gets in this condition and is morbidly obese, surgeons can remove part of the stomach or staple part of it shut. The patient feels full with smaller meals but must eat six or more meals a day and take many supplements. This drastic surgery can have side effects like diarrhea since fewer digestive enzymes are produced. It should be considered only as a last resort.

Fat distribution can be predetermined by your body type based on heredity

One woman might have big breasts. Another will have fat around her hips, no matter how much weight she loses. Advertisements showing women with thin thighs can be destructive to a healthy body image. Some women never get thin thighs despite losing other body fat.

As mentioned earlier, I went on a diet because I started getting fat on my hips and thighs. Even when I went from 123 pounds to 102 pounds, I could never get the 18-inch thighs I wanted. Meanwhile, I was always cold as my body tried to retain the few calories I gave it. In fact, my metabolism is still low, despite the many years between then and now. My extreme diet had a lasting negative effect. Even though thyroid tests show I'm in the low normal range, my basal temperature is lower than average and I feel cold in a room others find comfortable.

Many young women become anorexic trying to take off the body fat determined by their female hormones. For healthy old age, the young must start with a realistic ideal body image. Age also makes a difference in fat. Since muscle is eight times as dense as fat, even a person of medium build may weigh less but have more fat as he or she ages. Twenty years ago, my weight varied between 120 and 124 pounds. Now it's between 116 and 120, but I can't wear some of the clothes I did then. I have less muscle but more fat. I need more strenuous exercise to regain muscle weight.

Most of the calories used by the body are to maintain the internal temperature

The normal is 98.6 degrees Fahrenheit. This correlates with the basal metabolism and is measured when a person is lying down. In general, a taller person has a higher Basal Metabolic Rate because with greater height, there is proportionately more skin surface to transfer heat from the body to the outside. Someone tall can be naturally slim. A fat person needs fewer calories to maintain a normal body temperature. That person is carrying around a built-in blanket. Moreover, as fat accumulates, the person doesn't want to move as much, further decreasing the number of food calories necessary. You can believe the obese person who says, "I hardly eat a thing but I still can't lose weight." She is not lying or eating in secret. She just doesn't need much food to maintain the basal temperature of her well-insulated body. Also, with little exercise she uses few additional calories for movement.

It is possible to modify your hereditary shape

Although a person can have a certain shape because of heredity, diet and exercise can modify it a great deal. In the Eades' book, *Protein Power*, are four pictures of the same man taken in a five-year period. He looks like four different people. The first photo shows him at age 43 when he was running 50 miles a week. He looked emaciated despite his high carbohydrate diet. He had many minor illnesses, indicating he was damaging his immune system. Two years later, he stopped running but still got most of his calories from carbohydrates. He then looked like many Americans, obviously obese. The third picture showed him with massive muscles after months on a high-protein diet connected with an intensive body building program. The last picture showed him with medium muscles that he can maintain without spending many hours either running or working out in the gym. He has reached the normal weight and proportions he can keep the rest of his life.

What is obesity?

The present definition of obesity is one factor driving healthy persons of medium body size to get thin. Thirty percent more than normal, not 20 percent, could be called obese. This should be based on body fat, not total weight, since a pound of muscle is eight times as dense as a pound of fat and metabolizes at a rate many times that of fat. One author says that a pound of fat uses two calories an hour while a pound of muscle uses 32 calories an hour at rest and more when moving. Others state that there is a 10-fold difference between fat and muscle metabolism.

It would be better to be realistic as to who is obese or over-weight? Medium-weight people are being coerced into trying to be thin. They account for a large proportion of dieters. When they fail using one system, they are candidates for other diets, potions and pills and may end up truly obese instead of being content as a healthy medium.

Studies that seem to link obesity to heart disease, cancer and diabetes ignore causes of the obesity

Native peoples in Arctic areas who look fat have lived for millennia on meat and fat but don't get metabolic diseases until they adopt a Western diet. Similarly, Polynesians who gained weight from eating pork, coconuts and yams remained healthy. Fat chiefs even had more status. Sumo wrestlers look grossly obese but aren't at risk as long as they eat like their ancestors.

Certain Native American tribes eating corn, squash and beans might have been plump but got fatter on a modern diet and many got diabetes. After centuries on a high-fiber diet, they don't tolerate sweet drinks, alcohol and other refined carbohydrates.

Most doctors think that obesity itself causes disease instead of it being an indicator of a bad diet and sedentary lifestyle. Studies show that some obese people no longer have diabetes or have less risk of a heart attack after losing only a few pounds. It tells me they stopped eating sugars and started exercising in order to lose that weight. It was not that less body fat made them healthier. Changing your lifestyle improves your health. Losing fat by liposuction helps only your appearance.

How do you keep track of your progress if you start a program to lose body fat?

In the 1950s and 1960s, books and articles told dieters to weigh themselves daily and keep a diary of all calories consumed. It made people obsessive about their weight and it didn't work. When they lowered their calories too much, they lost muscle tissue and water. This showed immediate results on the scales, but couldn't last. People became discouraged when they hit a plateau and the scales showed the same weight for many days, despite the continual hunger pangs from the meager diet. They added more food but the scales showed the same number. Then they realized they looked fatter despite the lower weight. They had gained fat but had not regained the depleted muscle tissue.

Sensible programs such as Weight Watchers urged people to lose more slowly and weigh once a week. This still required counting calories or eating special dinners. Drs. Rachael and Richard Heller in *The Carbohydrate Addicts Diet* say to weigh daily then average this to find out what you have lost for the week. Dr. Henry Chang in *Weight Lost Forever* has his patients weigh every day. Frequent weighing is not appropriate for most people.

Many dieters are still fixated on the numbers on the scales and think that just losing weight makes them healthy. After you start exercising and improving your diet, instead of seeing if you have lost pounds, see if you have permanently lost inches from your body. Body wraps that just compress fat or flabby tissues is only temporary.

It is important to have lower measurements rather than fewer pounds

Muscle weighs more than fat so scales can be deceiving. A friend in a small town northeast of London belonged to a group trying to lose fat. She said they used the term "slimming" rather than "losing weight." It's a sensible idea probably related to the old way of expressing weight in *stones*. Since one stone is equivalent to 14 pounds, someone who says she weighs eight stones might be somewhere between 112 and 126 pounds. After all, a person can build muscle and be slimmer but weigh the same or even more than before. Weight can vary from day to day depending on the amount of salt in your diet or if you retain water before a menstrual period.

In the chapter on Allergies and Addictions, you'll learn that if your body can't tolerate certain foods you get "false fat." This is from extra fluids in your body tissues that make you weigh more and can cause abdominal bloating.

Look honestly at your own particular dimensions and frame. Be the best you can be, using healthy, natural means. Trying to get thin has made many millions of Americans fat using unhealthy crash diets. These always have a rebound effect so you get less healthy as well as fatter.

Don't get carried away by numbers, whether it's weight or dimensions or percentage of body fat. You want to be healthy, no matter what the numbers. After using any of the methods above, decide what your ideal healthy weight or body dimensions could be. Then comes the hard part –finding the diet or exercise program that's best for you. I'll present several from books or research articles, often based on differing premises. Ideal health as you get older is the goal and body fat is just one of the indicators. A specific weight is not an end in itself.

I would say a healthy woman should have between 20 percent and 30 percent body fat and a man should have between 13 percent and 20 percent fat. As mentioned earlier, this is not the same as Body Mass Index. A BMI of 20-22 is ideal, 22-25 still healthy, 25-30 is overweight and more than 30 is obese, disregarding the exceptions mentioned earlier.

Don't try to get thin

Don't get fat but aim for the Golden Mean of a healthy, age-defying medium weight that's right for you.

What You Can Do:

- Establish a baseline of your weight. The lowest is probably just after waking up and before break-fast. Weigh yourself again on two other days and average them.

- Figure out your Body Mass Index using the for-mula or from a chart on the internet.

- Get your approximate amount of body fat by floating in a pool or seeing if you can pinch more than an inch of fat in several places.

- Take your measurements at this time, holding the tape snug but not tight. The most important for both men and women is the waist measurement taken at the level of the navel. Women can also measure bust, hips and thighs while standing tall. Other measurements can include the chest below your breasts and the abdomen half-way between your waist and hips.

- Don't weigh yourself more than once a month. Do it at the same time of day and on the same day of your menstrual cycle. It's usually lowest after the end of your period.

- Take your abdominal measurement. See if it has changed during that first month. Take other mea-surements every three months as you continue a healthy diet and exercise.

- Another way is to try on a favorite piece of clothing that used to fit. As you lose body fat you'll again be able to put it on.

- If you want to keep a diary, keep track of your daily amount of exercise whether it is miles walked or time spent in other movement.

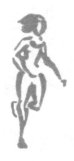

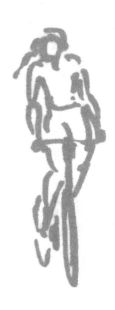

Myths &
Misinformation

Before looking at basic physiology and various diets and food programs, let's dispel a few long-standing myths and some that are promoted in print, on air or the Internet.

What you eat might not help your body. Unlike primitive men, we don't believe you can make your heart stronger by eating a powerful enemy's heart. Drinking red wine doesn't build up your blood even if it's the right color and was given for anemia for centuries. In the twentieth century certain foods were thought to help a part of the body which used a mineral that was in the food. Fish was called a brain food because it contains phosphorus and the brain has phospholipids. Oysters were considered good for male functions since they contain zinc as semen does. Other foods contain phosphorus or zinc and don't have any mystique.

Where does body fat come from?

It's a myth that the fat you eat goes directly into your fat cells, or that eating fat makes you fat. The Jack Sprat rhyme from our childhood is too simplistic. We don't know what else either he or his wife ate. If she were deficient in protein she might have craved sugars. In fact, both proteins and carbohydrates can be changed into fat and go into the fat cells. Since the Middle Ages, the French have produced tasty, high-fat goose-liver pâté from geese tied to a stake. These birds got no exercise and had nothing to do but eat carbohydrate-filled grain. Most of us aren't farmers, so we don't know that eating lots of grain can make an animal fat if it doesn't get enough exercise. Even when given protein-rich soybeans in the feed lots, steers don't gain more muscle - only fat.

Liquids can end up as fat. The fattest people I know get most of their calories not from fats or starchy or sweet foods but from sweet liquids. Worst are the cola addicts who drink six or more cans a day. Caffeine in the cola as well as the sugar causes a spike in insulin production. This can produce light-headedness and the desire for more sugar, satisfied by another can of soda pop. People who think they're being healthy by drinking lots of orange juice when they're hungry are getting many sugar calories. A dentist told his patients to boil down a quart of orange juice and see the syrup that results. Too much orange juice can produce body fat. Since it doesn't have fiber, you drink too much, often the equivalent of four to six oranges. If you ate the whole fruit, you would feel satisfied with one or two oranges and thus get fewer calories.

Alcohol can keep a body fat. Alex says he eats very little but can't lose weight. He doesn't count the calories in his two or three martinis a day. Alcohol is a molecule that cannot be made into the blood sugar needed by the brain. It becomes fat or is burned as fuel to keep the body temperature up. Alcohol has about seven calories per gram, intermediate between that of carbohydrates at four and fat at nine calories.

Some authors give misinformation about yeast

Carol had just recovered from a vaginal yeast infection and never wanted another. Someone told her to avoid dietary yeast and any product made by yeast. Food yeast is *Saccharomyses*, the good organism that helps bread to rise. Related yeasts ferment grain into beer or fruit into wine. The yeast that causes disease is *Candida*, a very different organism that can cause vaginal infections or overgrow in the intestines. These two types of yeast are as different as men are from mice. Rather than avoiding foods made with yeast, Carol should avoid sugar since *Candida* yeast thrives when a person's blood sugar gets too high. One author states that brewer's yeast is a nasty by-product of the beer industry foisted on humans. Some yeast is bitter but that in most health food stores has a delicious nutty flavor. It is specially grown in media to add trace minerals such as selenium and chromium in a very usable form. In addition yeast has natural proteins and B vitamins.

Acid-tasting foods rarely make your body acidic

Back in the 1920s, when the concept of pH became widespread, people worried whether a food was acidic or basic. Many myths persist even with increased knowledge about the breakdown of foods in the digestive system and their use within the cells. Something might test acidic or taste sour but it won't make the body acidic. Citrus fruits and tomatoes are sour but most of their organic acids break down within the body to water and carbon dioxide. Other acids with a benzene ring, like that in cranberry juice, retain their acidity as they go through the body, so are useful in treating bladder infections. Excess ascorbic acid (vitamin C) can also be excreted unchanged in the urine.

An acid reaction within the body is often from meat and soft drinks. Meat contains phosphates, sulfates and nitrates. Most soft drinks have phosphoric acid. All these fixed acids stay acidic in the body and in the urine. However, most amino acids formed by the breakdown of proteins don't stay acidic. When NH3 radicals are removed and excreted as urea, the resultant molecules are metabolized like carbohydrates into carbon dioxide and water. Diet books that make you worry about the acids in fruit or tomatoes are just plain wrong.

pH and stomach acid

Years ago an advertisement for a brand of coffee said, "Ours is acid-neutralized so you don't get that bitter acid taste." Anything bitter would have a basic, not an acidic reaction. A pH of 7 is neutral like water so is neither sour (acidic) nor bitter (basic). Anything below 7 is acidic and above 7 is basic. The pH scale is like the Richter scale for earthquakes, so pH 6 is 10 times as acidic; pH 5 is 100 times as acidic, like some fruit juices. Vinegar has an even lower pH. The hydrochloric acid produced in your stomach is about pH 2 or about 100,000 times as acidic as water.

The acid produced by cells in the stomach because of the caffeine in coffee might give you heartburn or acid reflux. This could also happen from caffeine-containing cola beverages. Alcohol and nicotine also cause your stomach to make more acid. The tomato juice in a Bloody Mary would not affect your stomach but the alcohol would increase its acid production. Smoking cigarettes while drinking black coffee or alcohol spells double-trouble for your stomach and esophagus because of the increased acid produced. Protect yourself by having food with your alcohol. Add cream to your coffee or have food when you drink it. Then you might not need a purple pill or an anti-acid.

Smoking was considered a relaxing habit in previous centuries and even today

Later, even when the connection with heart disease and lung cancer was known, people smoked to enhance their sex appeal. Men want to seem more masculine and women smoke to be thinner. Many people became chain smokers, never being without their favorite brand. I remember one four-pack-a-day friend with the rugged looks of the Marlboro Man. However, when I squeezed his arm, it wasn't firm but felt like soft putty. I assume he became one of the half-million people who die every year from smoking-related illnesses.

Heart disease is more common than lung cancer in both men and women. Nicotine causes small blood vessels to clamp down. If a coronary artery in the heart constricts, it causes the pain of angina. If vessels in a pregnant woman's uterus constrict, less blood gets through to her growing baby – one cause of small or premature babies. When the vessels in a person's skin constrict, collagen is damaged, causing sagging and early wrinkles. Young women who smoke to be thin like the movie stars they idolize don't realize that these smoking sirens needed cosmetic surgery to tighten the skin ravaged by nicotine.

Urine is not just from what you drink

A child thinks a little tube goes from the stomach to the bladder. In a 150-pound man, 190 quarts of liquid go from his blood through his kidneys every day. Most of it is reabsorbed back into the blood; only 2 quarts of liquid, along with urea, uric acid and some minerals, go into his bladder. Coffee, tea and alcohol affect the kidneys indirectly by causing capillaries in the kidneys to take out more liquid and direct this excess into the bladder making a larger amount of more dilute urine.

One acquaintance who says she's a caffeine addict thought that a spoonful of dehydrated coffee could give her the desired zip without the urge to empty her bladder on a long trip. The little water in a cup of coffee is not what gets into her bladder. It's the caffeine that causes more liquid to go through the kidneys into the bladder. Another acquaintance thought that if he drank martinis instead of beer at a party, he wouldn't have excess urine. This was harder on him than being the "middle-man for a golden liquid." As the alcohol stimulated the kidneys to excrete more urine, the liquid had to come from all his body tissues, causing dehydration worse than being in a desert.

Seeds and fiber

A long-standing myth warns against swallowing seeds. As a child, I heard some bad news. The father of a classmate had died of appendicitis, according to a neighbor who related the information to my mother. Mr. Jones always had some constipation but this time it lasted three or four days. Taking extra laxatives didn't help. He got pain in his right side and then a fever. That night his wife called the doctor who said he might need an operation. Mr. Jones knew he didn't have the money to go to the hospital but thought a hot-water bottle and aspirin would help. The next morning when she saw her husband paralyzed by pain, his wife got a neighbor to take him to the hospital. The doctor removed his swollen appendix successfully but the patient died a few hours later. The doctor said there were several grape seeds in the appendix. Everyone assumed the seeds must have caused the appendicitis so they told their children not to swallow any kind of seed.

Before the discovery of antibiotics, some doctors removed a

healthy appendix in connection with any abdominal operation to prevent a future problem. The appendix is like the uninflated end of a balloon and serves no purpose in humans. In dogs or other animals this is a fully inflated caecum where the small intestine dumps into the large intestine. In the past, most doctors suggested that vegetables be well cooked and seeds be removed from all fruits and vegetables.

In fact starting in the 1920s, soft, pure diets with little roughage caused many appendicitis attacks. The bowel acted slowly and because of this seeds sometimes got into the blind-ended appendix along with fecal material. Unhealthy chemicals made by certain bacteria stayed a long time in the gut. With high-fiber diets, there is enough action that seeds pass through and don't remain - even in the appendix. While some older recipes advocate removing the soft seeds of cucumbers, peppers and tomatoes as well as harder ones, I see no need to avoid seeds.

Modern low-fiber diets cause colitis as well as appendicitis

Fiber and seeds are a healthy and natural part of fresh fruits and vegetables. The fiber in these foods does not cause disease but prevents it. Formerly called roughage, cellulose is one type of fiber. Some authors make their readers think fruits are best drunk as juice and vegetables should be pulverized in a food processor. At least most of these are raw, but they don't give the intestine enough to work on. Persons with the smallest bowel movements are more likely to have cancer of the intestine. Toxins made by some bacteria in a high meat diet can weaken the gut lining. When a constipated person strains, he might cause outpouching called diverticulae like tiny appendices. If these collect fecal matter and get infected, painful diverticulitis can result.

Mildred had been told to avoid all raw fruits and vegetables because she had colitis. Her soft diet had probably caused this problem. When she strained during defecation she caused the pouches of diverticulosis. Feces collected and certain bacteria increased too much, causing inflammation. With no second opinion, Mildred persisted with the same diet. Her husband, who started eating this low-fiber diet, also developed what the doctor called colitis. Later, Mildred had symptoms of folic acid deficiency from the lack of fresh fruits and vegetables. She takes folic acid pills but keeps her soft diet accompanied by chemical laxatives. She could have avoided the problem by having enough fruits and vegetables, both cooked and raw, all of her life. If you eat enough fiber, your intestinal contents, including seeds and bacteria, move rapidly without harm. Our ancestors and the primitive peoples of today eat whole raw fruits and vegetables.

Effects of fiber

Dr. T.L. Cleave, a surgeon-captain in the British Royal Navy, researched the effect of fiber. He says it takes more than 30 years for diverticulosis to develop. According to Dr. Cleave, the prevalence of this condition correlates better with heart disease than does eating animal fat. He noted that from 1900 to 1970, the consumption of fat had increased very little but most Westerners ate fewer high-fiber foods. Even in the past 30 years, as some people consumed less fat, they didn't add more fiber.

One survey in the early 2000's showed that the average family of four spent only $3 to $4 a week on fresh produce. That might buy a head of lettuce, some carrots and apples. My grocery cart contains mostly vegetables, some fresh fruit, frozen berries and pineapple. I might buy a jar of unsweetened applesauce but no juices.

More than 30 years ago, Dr. Sanford Siegal promoted his natural fiber permanent weight loss diet. Dr. Siegal mentions studies where Zulus gave up their high-fiber diet and ate modern diets. Conditions unknown to tribal peoples such as cancer, diabetes and heart disease, as well as colitis and diverticulosis, occurred with the modern foods.

What can we learn from this? Natural foods have two types of fiber. **Insoluble fiber**, also known as cellulose or roughage, can't be digested by humans. Only herbivores have special bacteria in their digestive tracts that break down cellulose to make carbohydrates and proteins these grazing animals can use. In humans and other omnivores, the insoluble fiber stimulates the action of the intestines to move digestive products and wastes. *Soluble fiber*, including pectins and lignins, is now well known. Pectin absorbs water and keeps the stools soft. Apples are high in pectin. Maybe by preventing constipation we got the saying "An apple a day keeps the doctor away." The most advertised soluble fiber is in oat bran since it absorbs cholesterol in the intestine and carries it out with the feces.

Over-processed foods:

Too many cultures act as though the purer and whiter a food is, the better. Some of this was because whole-grains were more likely to attract weevils and other insects. Therefore, even the poor farmers in Southeast Asia winnow their rice to blow off the chaff and get a white product. They throw away the nutritious germ of the grain along with the mineral-rich husk. White sugar and white flour, just like white rice, can be stored for a long time without spoiling. They contain carbohydrates but none of the minerals and vitamins originally present. Is a long shelf-life really a desirable trait?

Recent studies show a similarity in the DNA of mammals and many lower forms of life: All cells that require oxygen have some of the same internal biochemistry, whether from bacteria, fungi, worms, insects or man. If a food can't support rapid growth of lower forms of life, it won't have all the vitamins and minerals to promote optimum growth and functioning of humans. You stay alive but don't have radiant good health.

Some weight loss programs have artificial formulas that include protein supplements. They taste like milk shakes and might have the protein, vitamins and minerals necessary for health, but contain too much sugar. Use them only as a temporary substitute for a good high-fiber meal that has antioxidants and other micro-nutrients. Even bottled smoothies often have a long list of artificial chemicals and high sugar content, along with a small amount of some natural fruit.

Do people prefer low-fiber foods? A Chinese woman imprisoned during the 10-year Cultural Revolution complained she didn't get enough white rice. But the yams and cabbage soup they fed her kept her alive better than rice would have. Similarly, even small 4-ounce pieces of heavy black bread many Russians got during the siege of Leningrad had more nutrients than could be found in white bread. However, Russians today prefer fresh crusty white bread. In 1993, I saw old women eking out a living by selling subsidized loaves of white bread to subway passengers. At least this white bread is superior to the soft, spongy bread Americans have been eating for more than 70 years. Maybe grade school kids like it because it's easy to chew when they're losing their baby teeth. Even when iron and some vitamins are added back, this white, spongy bread is inferior to whole-grain bread containing natural vitamins and fiber.

Raw foods

Eating only raw foods might be going too far. One doctor blames all the ills of civilization on cooked food. He says the enzymes in raw foods partially digest the food itself. The rest then become the enzymes of your body cells. In fact, only raw pineapple and raw papaya have digestive enzymes. They can be used in marinades as a tenderizer. Once eaten, these enzymes are soon destroyed.

Raw food advocates base their theory on a 1940s study by Dr. Francis M. Pottenger that focused on the diet of 900 cats. They all got the same minimal diet. In addition, one group had raw milk, another got raw meat products. They and their kittens stayed healthy. Other groups got processed foods and heated milk that was pasteurized, evaporated or condensed. They developed cancer and diabetes in old age. Their offspring got these diseases in middle age. The next descendents of the "heated-food cats" were abnormal even as kittens. They wouldn't play or fight, did not have the normal righting reflex when dropped upside-down and later couldn't reproduce.

However, there are problems with citing this study as the reason to eat only raw foods. Information is missing. Other foods in the minimal basic diet weren't described nor were other factors.

What utensils were used? Was the pasteurized or canned milk from a reputable manufacturer? Maybe lead was used in sealing the cans. Such drastic symptoms suggest that heavy metal poisoning must have caused the extreme metabolic problems in the "heated-food cats."

This is similar to a report a few years back of third graders in a nutrition study. They raised pairs of rats, feeding some on cookies and doughnuts and others on seeds or grain. One boy said that his rat who got doughnuts was still okay but the one who got seeds started getting convulsions in a couple of weeks and died. I suspect the boy used packets of seeds meant for planting. Many of these are dusted with a mercury compound to prevent fungi from attacking their tender roots just after germination. The rat probably died of mercury poisoning.

Most natural foods do not form toxins when cooked; some require cooking to destroy toxins

Legumes like beans and lentils contain substances that become harmless only *after cooking.* Raw lima beans have caused death and uncooked fava beans can produce hemolytic anemia according to Dr. Carl Pfeiffer in *Mental and Elemental Nutrients.* He also says that eating the pea-like seeds or dry, ground meal from vetches has caused paralysis in people in Europe, Africa and Asia. Common white mushrooms are okay to eat raw, but most other edible mushrooms need cooking. When I tried raw crimini mushrooms, I got stomach cramps. Cooked ones caused no problem. Fruit, vegetables and whole-grains are better for you than manufactured foods but some natural foods must be cooked.

Raw foods do contain enzymes. Enzymes are proteins whose molecules are folded in a specific way to get other molecules together to react. They are inactivated by heat, which disrupts this complex folding. Like other proteins, most enzymes are also degraded by the acid produced in the stomach. Ethnic groups treat raw fish with vinegar or lemon juice to mimic the effect of cooking. Enzymes are broken down like other proteins in your stomach and intestines. These very large molecules can't be absorbed intact into your blood stream to go into your body tissues. Your body cells make their own enzymes from amino acids in a healthy diet. Fresh raw foods are beneficial but not because of the enzymes within their cells.

Sometimes toxins can be formed in cooked food. Foods subjected to very high temperatures do form undesirable products. Formerly healthy fats, proteins or even carbohydrates can be changed and oxidized to a less healthy form. Purists say never to eat anything barbecued or deep-fried and even stay away from Liquid Smoke. In reality, a healthy person's liver can neutralize most of these toxins as long as it isn't overloaded. Only occasionally eat well-browned or deep-fried meat or french fries and enjoy them as a special treat.

One friend is so worried about the changes in browned food that he never eats dark brown toast. However, he drinks a lot of Scotch whiskey. The amber color and flavor of any whiskey comes from being aged in charred oak barrels and Scotch also has burnt peat. These substances that come from subjecting wood to fire are much more damaging than dark brown toast. This is an example of selective awareness.

Toxins within the body

According to some diet books, fasting removes toxins from your body. They say that after fasting for several days you will notice your urine is darker from excreted toxins and your breath smells bad. This supposedly shows that fasting lets your body get rid of these toxins.

In reality, the fast itself caused these chemicals to be formed from your muscles and body fat. Since the body has no food from which to make blood glucose for the brain, it first uses up the limited store of glycogen in your liver and muscles. Later, it has to break down body proteins by removing the NH3 groups from amino acids to produce carbohydrate intermediates. These amino groups then combine with carbon dioxide to be excreted as urea in your urine.

The body also breaks down fats. It burns them two molecules

at a time as active acetate, leaving residual molecules that form ketone bodies. Some of these are excreted in the urine. Others are breathed out as acetone. Fasting causes these break-down products to be formed in large quantities from your own healthy muscle and fat. The fast itself produced the toxins. They can be diluted by drinking lots of water but wouldn't it be better not to form them in the first place?

Do the intestines need cleaning?

Some myths say we have to cleanse our intestines by using enemas to wash out the accumulated toxins, especially from animal products since they take too long to be defecated and might get into our blood. They say the intestinal tracts of carnivores are short to get rid of toxic products quickly. In reality, they are shorter because animal products are digested more easily than that of a diet containing plant foods. Herbivores need to retain their fibrous vegetable food longer to give the special bacteria in their digestive tract time to break it down. Humans have moderately long intestines, as do other omnivores. We have enzymes in the stomach and small intestine that break down proteins, fats and carbohydrates. We just can't use cellulose for food. This insoluble fiber is necessary only to promote regularity.

Some people claim there can be pounds of fecal matter in our colons that remain there to fester for weeks, months or years. It would be unusual for anyone to retain pounds of fecal matter. If you did it would require surgery to remove the large impacted lumps. Besides being acted upon by digestive enzymes, part of the intestinal contents is food for beneficial bacteria that produce certain vitamins. The small intestine is self-cleansing. New intestinal cells mature every day and push the older cells off into the intestine forming about a third of your feces. Almost a third is bacteria and the rest is the indigestible fiber from your food. You don't need high colonic enemas to wash these substances out. They are normal. Besides eating insoluble fiber from bran or vegetables to keep your intestines active, it is good to drink enough water to keep your stools soft. This is most important on a long drive through the desert or on long airline flights where the air is very dry.

The toxins to worry about are those from disease-causing bacteria. Examples are salmonella from under-cooked chicken and certain types of *E. coli* from under-done hamburger. The body reacts to the toxins from these bacteria or from some viruses and tries to get rid of them. If you try to stop this action with a chemical, the bacteria and their products stay in your intestine longer. Kaopectate was good for moderate diarrhea since the kaolin clay absorbed the toxins and the pectin absorbed excess liquid. It seems this combination is no longer manufactured. You can get Pepto-Bismol world-wide but it is less benign and can kill helpful bacteria as well as the harmful ones. Any antibiotic you take could also kill your beneficial bacteria and allow a yeast infection to start. Applesauce is good to normalize intestinal function when there aren't dangerous bacteria. Its pectin absorbs the excess water of mild diarrhea.

Environmental toxins are another matter. It would be hard to get these out of your system by drinking excess water or using enemas. Heavy metals such as lead can be removed in a hospital with injections of a chelating agent such as EDTA (ethylene diamine tetra-acetic acid). In a later chapter I'll discuss antioxidants and vitamins that help your liver to neutralize some of the organic toxins.

Oxygen

Some people say to breathe deeply to get more oxygen to all your cells. Maybe they remember the old saying from school health classes, "We inhale oxygen and exhale carbon dioxide." When you're sedentary, your cells use less than one-fifth of the oxygen in your blood. The large amount of unused oxygen you breathe out makes mouth-to-mouth resuscitation possible. Even during strenuous aerobic exercise, an average person uses only about 75 percent of the available oxygen for his or her active muscles and the faster beating heart.

The body does not get more oxygen from deep breathing. Swimmers who think they can "charge their blood with oxygen" by taking many deep breaths aren't getting more into their blood cells. The reason they can swim longer under water is they have blown off excess carbon dioxide and don't have the urge to breathe that comes with too much carbon dioxide rather than too little oxygen in the blood.

If you hike at high altitudes, you don't get more oxygen by breathing harder. Take slow breaths to let your body absorb the oxygen you have in your lungs & blood. Fast breathing again blows off too much carbon dioxide. This disrupts the balance of carbonic acid and other acids and minerals in your blood stream and might cause altitude sickness.

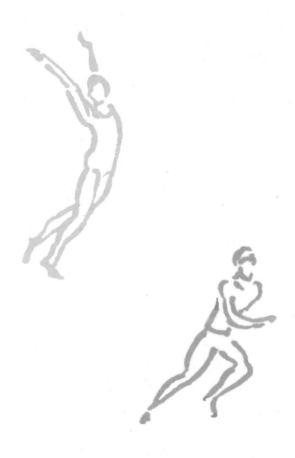

Summary

- Body fat can be formed from any food or alcohol, but most easily from sugars and starches.

- Dietary yeast and the foods made with it do not cause yeast infections in the body.

- Most acid-tasting foods do not cause the body to be more acidic. Only complex acids like that in cranberry juice make your urine acidic. Meat and most soft drinks can cause an acid reaction.

- Caffeine, alcohol and nicotine can cause the stomach to produce too much acid.

- Tobacco use is not glamorous.

- Coffee, tea or alcohol can cause the kidneys to send more urine to the bladder.

- Fiber is necessary for healthy intestinal functions. Use whole-grain products and plenty of fruits and vegetables. Don't worry about seeds.

- Most raw foods are good for you, but your body makes its own enzymes.

- Foods subjected to very high temperatures can contain less healthy products.

- Fasting does not cleanse the body of toxins. Fasting produces toxins.

- It is unnecessary to cleanse the intestine with enemas or the kidneys with excess water.

- Deep breathing doesn't put extra oxygen into your cells.

Basic Chemistry & Physiology

Before we look at healthy diets, you need to know more about how the cells and organ systems in your body work. Some of the chapters are complex and introduce many new words. Skip them for now, but they are essential in understanding the diets that have caused more obesity and metabolic diseases in the past thirty years.

During recent years, a low-fat, no-cholesterol, high-carbohydrate diet has been touted by the media and accepted as gospel by the majority of Americans. Meanwhile, heart disease has increased even though people have been eating much less cholesterol and saturated fat. The number of fat people has more than doubled and more people have diabetes. In the following chapters you will read about several doctors and others who dispute the commonly accepted theories about the dangers of saturated fat and cholesterol. The chapter on cardiovascular disease will show other factors that cause atherosclerosis.

Doctors are cautious and don't readily accept new theories. Standard medical ideas do change, but it might take many years. Drs. Wilfred and Evan Shute of Canada claimed in the 1950s that taking Vitamin E helps the heart and blood vessels. Years later, almost everyone agrees it's good for general health as well as for the heart. Dr. Sanford Siegal in the 1970s veered from standard thought by stating that fiber was essential to health. Now the medical establishment says to eat more fiber. For more than 30 years, Dr. John Yudkin has been saying that use of refined sugar is related to cardiovascular disease. Most doctors ignored his book *Sweet and Dangerous.* Many still say the only thing wrong with sugar is it can rot your teeth. Unless there is an incentive to produce a new expensive pill, basic research testing a new theory won't be funded. Russel Reiter, Ph.D. in his book *Melatonin* says that is true of the natural hormone melatonin, as well as other substances. Drs. Michael and Mary Dan Eades in *The Protein Power Life Plan* in a chapter on magnesium tell how this mineral could replace many expensive medications. Since it can't be patented, no drug company is interested in doing research on magnesium.

The weight-loss industry and the manufactured food industry accept new ideas more quickly. If profits can be made, industry will come out with products that cater to any fad. Now that thousands of Americans are on the low-carbohydrate, high-protein Atkins diet, many new "low- carb." packaged foods are appearing in the grocery stores.

You can be skeptical and not be swayed either by the medical-pharmaceutical industry or advocates of fad diets. Respect the wisdom of the human body to heal itself as you learn more about how it works. You can ignore theories that apply only to certain groups of people even if some media reporters imply that everyone should follow the same suggestions. One size does not fit all.

Some Facts About Basic Chemistry & Physiology

The body is not a chemical vat

Laymen and some authors assume all you need to do is consume the food, mineral or other substance and it goes where you think it should to make you healthy. That's not always the case. Reactions inside the cells are complex. They differ depending on whether the cell is in the liver, the brain, muscles, intestines or fat deposits. Even interactions of cells by way of chemical messengers in the blood might not be perfect in some people.

Many reactions respond to automatic feedback. If you form

more of a metabolic product than you need, the excess shuts down the reaction so no more is made for awhile. The reactants then go down an alternative pathway to make something else or be excreted. Many reactions can go in either direction. Combine two substances and get a product. But if you take more of the product as a supplement, it might cause the reaction to go backward. Instead of getting additional amounts of something, your body might get rid of more of what you have as it goes down a different chemical pathway. Some reactions can't go backwards because energy was released in the formation of a product. This is true when glucose is metabolized by a long series of steps to pyruvic acid and then to active-acetate, the important source of energy in most cells. Active-acetate can also be made into cholesterol or fat but not glycogen or blood sugar.

Your body might not absorb what you take in

Taking minerals, vitamins or other substances might not be very effective. Your body might be missing vitamins or trace minerals that enhance the action of vitamins. A substance in your diet can block the absorption of a dietary supplement. For example, some people can't absorb extra iron even if it is needed so the extra iron goes out in the feces as iron sulfide. You might have noticed that you get black stools when you take iron pills. The section on minerals tells more about iron metabolism.

You need stress on your bones to signal the need for more calcium. If you're sedentary, calcium can go through the gut unabsorbed. One doctor was mystified by half-inch-long opaque objects in the x-rays of the intestines of some of his patients. These were calcium pills that hadn't dissolved even in the high acidity of the stomach. Even well-chewed calcium pills might not put calcium into your bones. Many older women have osteoporosis, a condition where their bones have lost calcium. Obese women are less likely to have osteoporosis because their heavy weight exerts a stress that keeps calcium in their bones.

You need certain amounts of minerals whether from food, pills or

liquids

Phosphorus must be in the correct ratio with calcium in your blood or calcium can come out of your bones. Magnesium must also be in proper balance with calcium. To keep the correct ratio of calcium to magnesium in your blood you need magnesium from pills, water or green vegetables. You need the sodium in salt to help keep water in your blood and tissues. A moderate excess goes out in urine. However, if you use too much salt, your body tries to dilute it by keeping more water in your body. This can cause ankle swelling or high blood pressure in some people.

The human body has evolved over eons so it can make most of the chemicals it needs

If you give your body the right raw materials from healthy food and proper exercise, it responds in a healthy manner. However, it can make blood glucose from any carbohydrate or protein, even those in junk foods. For good health you need vitamins, minerals, essential amino acids and essential fatty acids in your diet. These are best when made by various plants and animals.

Amino acids repair muscle cells or form enzymes, cell membranes and other body proteins. Essential amino acids are those that can't be made by the body but must come pre-formed from the diet. Similarly essential fatty acids must come from your diet to help form cell membranes and keep skin and joints healthy. Most vitamins act as co-enzymes (cofactor or helpers) of various enzymes to get energy out of food and to produce specialized cells. Green leafy vegetables contain the co-factor folic acid along with magnesium and other minerals. More about these substances will be found in the chapter on supplements.

Antioxidants are a diverse group of molecules

Some are made within our cells, but many must come from food. We need some antioxidants to counteract pollutants in the air. Others counteract free radicals formed during many of the reactions inside our cells. Vitamin C is the best known, along with vitamins A and E. A common characteristic of antioxidants is the double bonds between two or more carbon atoms. These are unstable and can break open to attach to a rogue oxygen atom or a more complex free radical. Antioxidants, contained in foods produced from plants, have been in the diet of ancient humans for millennia. The bright yellow and orange of squash and carrots are evidence of carotenoids and the dark reds and blues in grapes and berries are from lycopenes. These and other substances show the value of eating lots of brightly colored fruits and vegetables.

Digestive enzymes act outside the cells, unlike enzymes within cells that need vitamins as co-factors

Digestive enzymes are secreted by special cells in the lining of the gastro-intestinal tract or from the pancreas to break down food in the stomach or intestine. Your salivary glands make an enzyme to start digesting starches. Most starch is digested later in the small intestine. The lining of the stomach contains a variety of glands. Some secrete hydrochloric acid that helps the enzyme pepsin, secreted by other cells, to start the breakdown of proteins in your diet to shorter units called peptides. The stomach protects itself with small glands in the lining that make a coating of mucus. Faulty diets, certain bacteria or some drugs can interfere with this self-protection, leading to ulcers.

The digestion of foods

Although fats and carbohydrates have a limited breakdown in the stomach, you can eat a mixture of foods at the same time. Proteins, carbohydrates and fats don't interfere with each other. Over eons of time, the digestive system has evolved to handle a variety of foods as they pass from the stomach down the three parts of the small intestine and into the colon.

After the contents of the stomach go into the small intestine, juices made in the pancreas join those from the gall bladder and go by a tube into the first part of the intestines, the duodenum. These juices contain mineral molecules that neutralize the strong stomach acid so pancreatic enzymes can finish the break-down of protein fragments to amino acids. Meanwhile, some pancreatic enzymes split off glucose molecules from carbohydrates and others help break down fats. Long-term abuse of alcohol can damage the pancreas so it can't produce these enzymes. This is as serious as cirrhosis of the liver caused by too much alcohol.

Fats, carbohydrates & sugars

Before looking at insulin and other hormones, the inter-relationships of some fats and sugars in cardiovascular disease and the body's reaction to stress, the following simple chemical definitions might help you:

Carbohydrates contain carbon atoms (C), each balanced by two hydrogen atoms (H) and the oxygen atom (O) in a ratio like that in water. The basic building block in carbohydrates is glucose, a six-carbon ring-shaped molecule. Starch is a chain of glucose molecules formed by plants. Glycogen is a chain or lattice of glucose molecules formed by animals. (Glucose is blood sugar.)

Fats contain only carbon (C) and hydrogen (H). Fatty acids are chains of carbon atoms usually with two hydrogen atoms attached to each. Three chains are attached to a three carbon molecule. The unsaturated fats have lost hydrogen atoms in specific places and have unstable carbon to carbon double bonds. These bonds easily open to react with oxygen. The resultant peroxides make the oil taste rancid or interfere with intra-cellular reactions.

Proteins contain nitrogen (N) as well as carbon, hydrogen and oxygen. Their basic building blocks are the amino acids. Some may contain sulfur. Proteins also may contain phosphates, nitrates or other mineral compounds. Protein molecules are very large, thousands of times larger than amino acids or glucose.

Enzymes are specialized proteins, folded in a specific way so they can aid chemical reactions. Simple enzymes act in the digestion of food. More complex ones are contained within all body cells to promote a variety of reactions to produce energy or to form other molecules.

Hormones are relatively small but complex molecules made in

one part of the body and carried by the blood to act in another part. Insulin is the best known.

Summary

- Give your body healthy natural foods and a moderate amount of extra vitamins and few other supplements. As long as you get enough exercise, your body will make all other cellular chemicals to keep you healthy without the necessity of expensive prescription pills.

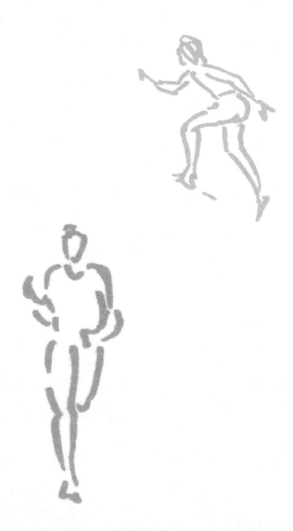

Maintaining Normal Insulin & Related Hormones

Certain cells in the pancreas regulate glucose by making two hormones, insulin and glucagon.

Hormones are chemicals formed in one part of the body that go via the blood vessels to act on another part of the body. When sugars from food or drink are absorbed, they cause cells in the pancreas to secrete insulin into the blood. This hormone brings the blood sugar back to normal levels by causing glucose molecules to enter cells all over the body. High blood sugar from eating sweets can make you feel good for a short time by increasing endorphins in the brain. Then insulin signals liver cells, muscle cells and fat cells to accept more sugar, some of which then becomes glycogen in liver and muscle cells. The rest becomes body fat. One reason a man can eat more sweets than a woman is that his bigger muscles can absorb more blood sugar, leaving less to go into fat cells.

During exercise, glucose can provide energy for the muscles. I have hiked with purists who won't let any sweets pass their lips even if their bodies are crying for some quick calories. Sugars can quickly enter the blood. Then insulin "opens the gates" into all body cells for glucose to enter. If you're sedentary, then most *glucose becomes fat.*

Trouble starts when blood sugar regulation is overactive and too much insulin is produced

When you consume too much sugar, your pancreas keeps making more insulin and your blood sugar drops too low, causing a condition called hypoglycemia. You might then relieve this weakness and light-headedness with another sugary snack. You get on a roller coaster of too high blood sugar followed by too much insulin followed by too low blood sugar then more sugar and more insulin. After several years the insulin receptors on the various glucose-accepting cells become damaged and they're resistant to the action of insulin. The blood sugar then stays too high, despite ever-higher levels of insulin. This causes adult-onset (type II) diabetes as the pancreas starts to fail. This is preceded by obesity and accompanied by cardiovascular disease.

Continued high insulin can cause injuries to the linings of many blood vessels

Cholesterol and fat are deposited to repair this damage. This can lead to coronary artery disease and kidney disease. Deposits in arteries to the brain might contribute to strokes. Many studies show high blood levels of insulin in these conditions, but the accompanying obesity or high cholesterol get the blame. Chronic high insulin is the real culprit, causing obesity and serious metabolic diseases. Some diabetics must avoid all sugars and the starches that the body easily converts to glucose. They are sugar addicts similar to alcoholics. Even a cookie can set some people off on a binge of more carbohydrates.

Glucagon, the other pancreatic hormone, antagonizes most natural functions of insulin

Its action is opposite to that of insulin. Instead of allowing glucose to go into cells, it causes the glycogen in muscle cells and the liver to break down into glucose and enter the blood stream. The action of glucagon restores the blood sugar to normal levels, not the extremely low levels caused by excess insulin. Glucagon also promotes the breakdown of fat into smaller molecules that go into the blood. Fat then gets used for energy. Heart muscle indeed prefers the molecules from fat breakdown as a concentrated form of energy. Only the brain requires glucose. During starvation, your body first uses glycogen to make glucose, then by an inefficient process uses molecules from the breakdown of muscles and fat to keep the brain functioning.

Insulin has other functions than making blood sugar available to all cells. Insulin can help get fat molecules from food out of the blood and into the tissues to use as energy or to store. Insulin stimulates the production of cholesterol in the liver. (As will be explained later, cholesterol is an indispensable component in cell membranes and is used in making the sex hormones.) Insulin causes the kidneys to retain salt and water producing higher blood pressure during greater physical exertion, just like adrenaline. A *moderate* amount of insulin causes small blood vessels to dilate to better carry blood to the tissues. Glucagon has an opposite effect in all these reactions and normalizes the body's physiology.

You can manipulate the glucagon/insulin ratio so it is appropriate for your body and activity level

Barry Sears, in his book *The Zone,* says to stimulate glucagon instead of insulin by eating more protein and fat. He recommends a diet with about 30 percent fat, 30 percent protein and 40 percent carbohydrate. Dietary protein does stimulate the production of glucagon, especially in the ratio of 3 parts protein to 4 parts carbohydrate, according to Sears.

Glucagon is ignored by advocates of extensive running. They say you can prevent high insulin spikes by eating complex carbohydrates that cause glucose to enter the blood more slowly than sugars. They also say never to get too hungry, but eat complex carbohydrates every couple of hours, then run some more. Even complex carbohydrates end up as glucose. I think it would make more sense to stimulate more glucagon.

Without mentioning glucagon, Dr. Robert Arnot says to snack on cooked soybeans rather than a grain product to get complex carbohydrates. Soybeans contain more protein then grains and almost twice as much protein as other beans. That would stimulate glucagon. Soybeans also have more fat, giving a feeling of satiety. Eating soybeans represents a middle way. Their balanced ratio of proteins, fats and carbohydrates can satisfy both vegetarians and omnivores. Other seeds and nuts have various ratios of protein, carbohydrate, fat and fiber. Though not as good as soybeans, these are superior in nutrients to packaged snack foods. Sunflower seeds have more fiber and carbohydrate than nuts, but like them contain some fat and protein to stimulate glucagon. The ads that say "Bet you can't eat just one" refer to potato chips, but it can apply to roasted, salted nuts. Roasted nuts with salt will stimulate the appetite for more salted nuts, leading you to reach for more. A few raw unsalted nuts can keep insulin down, activate glucagon and not add many calories.

Fat in the diet causes the body to make secretin, another hormone

As fats are partially digested in the duodenum, secretin and other hormones enter the blood stream to tell the brain to delay the emptying of the stomach. Therefore you don't get hungry again too soon. If you suffer from hypoglycemia (too low blood sugar) after eating carbohydrates, you should instead eat nuts or cheese. Their fat and protein activate secretin, elevate your glucagon level, don't cause elevated insulin and keep your blood sugar in a normal range. Meanwhile, glucagon stimulates the burning of fat for energy. This is much more effective in preventing hypoglycemia than eating complex carbohydrates.

Leptin is a hormone made by cells in body fat

After a certain amount of glucose enters fat cells to become fat, these cells in normal people make leptin, a satiety hormone. When leptin goes via the blood to a person's brain, he or she feels satisfied and stops eating. Leptin's action was first noted in a strain of very obese rats that lacked the gene that makes it. Many obese humans make plenty of leptin but are resistant to its action.

Insulin's actions become exaggerated and ultimately harmful when you consume too much sugar

As insulin levels rise and stay too high, this overrides the action of glucagon. When a person's cells don't react to insulin to take in blood sugar, this is called insulin-resistance. The high insulin levels cause blood vessels to go into spasm. Blood platelets then get sticky and form small clots. If blood pressure goes up, small blood vessels can be injured. This causes foam cells and cholesterol to collect at the site of the injury. Cholesterol is a necessary component of all cell membranes so the vessels are stimulated to form new smooth muscle cells to repair their injuries using cholesterol. Vessels might become stiffer, sometimes with a smaller inside diameter. These attempted repairs continue in other vessels as long as there is insulin-resistance.

Saying that the cholesterol that accumulates in the plaque caused the plaque to form is like saying that the bandages a first aid worker wraps around a wound to stop the bleeding caused the wound, or the patch you put on a tire produced the original flat. Doctors should look back on their pathology classes, where they saw slides of the thickening of blood vessels in the kidney and the deposits of fat and cholesterol in other vessels of diabetic patients. They would realize that high blood sugar and too-high insulin of obese diabetics were to blame, not *dietary* fats being deposited directly into the vessels. Insulin causes the liver to make cholesterol and fat from excess sugars and to release them into the blood. Avoiding cholesterol and fat in the diet won't prevent this.

Fructose was once thought to be a benign alternative to sucrose (table sugar).

Even 70 years ago, diabetes specialists used honey to keep their patients' blood glucose low so they wouldn't need as much insulin. Honey contains fructose and is twice as sweet as sucrose so you can use half as much. Since fructose can be metabolized by an alternative pathway instead of being transformed into glucose, it doesn't raise the blood sugar level or cause an increase in insulin. The amount of fructose in fruit is low at 2 to 7 percent and no cause for alarm. Honey has been used in small amounts over the centuries, with no apparent harm.

In the past 30 years, the use of high-fructose corn syrup as a sweetener has increased dramatically. Since it is cheaper than sucrose and more easily stored, manufacturers of soft drinks and makers of sweet, packaged products now use much more of it. People in the United States consume 16 billion pounds of high-fructose corn syrup each year, as reported by N.Y.U professor Marion Nestle in *Food Politics: How the Food Industry Influences Nutrition and Health.* That's more than 50 pounds per person. This represents a third or more of the 120 to 150 pounds of sweeteners the average American now eats or drinks per year. It is certainly adding to obesity in the U.S. Nestle states that 10 billion cases of soft drinks were consumed in the U.S. in 2001. This is about 53 gallons per person. If only half the people in the nation drink soft drinks, that amounts to more than a quart a day for each of them. The leading sellers were Classic Coke at 1.9 billion cases and Pepsi-Cola at 1.3 billion cases. These contain high-fructose corn syrup, not cane sugar.

Fructose might be more dangerous than sucrose

Dr. John Bantle of the University of Minnesota, reported in the November 1992 issue of the journal *Diabetes Care*, research on both type I and type II diabetics. Those who substituted fructose for glucose in their diets indeed did not have spikes in the levels of blood sugar or insulin. However, their cholesterol increased, especially the low density "bad" cholesterol. (The chapter on cardiovascular disease will tell more about this research.)

Diet drinks might cause other problems

Diet Coke and Diet Pepsi, at 879 million and 534 million cases respectively, are not entirely harmless. Even the supposedly safe chemical sweeteners in them might cause side effects. In the 1960s, cyclamates were used extensively in diet soft drinks. Betty, who had several cola drinks a day, changed to the diet varieties when she got pregnant so she wouldn't gain too much weight. She didn't connect the drinks with the fact that the fetus died at about the fourth month in that and a subsequent pregnancy. After a publicized report in an obscure Japanese journal that cyclamate caused fetal mice to die *in utero*, cyclamates were withdrawn. Then manufacturers went back to saccharine, a chemical sweetener introduced decades earlier. Betty didn't like the metallic aftertaste in these diet colas but carried her next pregnancy to term.

All non-caloric sweeteners should be used with caution. The caffeine in a diet soft drink can cause a rise in insulin in some people. An artificial sweetener makes you crave more sweets instead of less. If only something made with sucrose or fructose is available, then that's what you'll consume. It's best to gradually get rid of a sweet tooth. Then you can appreciate other flavors, like the tartness of many fruits. You won't be one of the millions of obese Americans addicted to sweets.

Besides making you fat, your sweet tooth can lead to excess insulin and later insulin resistance. The resultant type II diabetes can injure blood vessels and might cause a heart attack or stroke. Sugar and other simple carbohydrates, not fats, are the substances to cut back or avoid completely for good health. Get rid of the diabetes and you reduce the chance of fat-clogged arteries and meanwhile lose excess body fat.

If cancer runs in your family, consider the following anecdote:

In the 1980s, I got a phone call from Alice, a friend in her late forties. She had just been diagnosed with intestinal cancer and asked if I knew of a new pill, a magic bullet that might cure it. Her doctor said she needed more than simple surgery. If she got either radiation or anti-cancer drugs, she would feel sicker and even then the odds for a cure were poor.

"It's important to get as healthy as possible so you can withstand the treatment," I suggested. "I assume you're eating a good balanced diet and not drinking or smoking now."

"Well, I did give up drinking when my doctor made the same observation you did about my red palms," Alice said. "I'm trying to quit smoking but it's difficult. I don't feel like eating much but I do take vitamin pills and drink lots of lemonade."

"The liquid and the vitamins are good, but I hope you're not putting too much sugar in your lemonade," I said. "This might not be relevant, but 10 years ago I had three friends die of three different types of cancer in one year. One woman of 65 died of ovarian cancer. Another, age 60 died of liver cancer while the third died of breast cancer at age 55. The only thing they had in common was they each made their lemonade way too sweet. The sugar didn't cause their cancers but it could have made them grow too fast."

To her silence I added, "I wish I had good news. I can't even come to visit because I have a cold I wouldn't want to give you." I hung up the phone feeling helpless.

We now have statistics showing increased cancer with diabetes. Rapidly growing cancer cells take advantage of high blood sugar. Dr. Bob Arnot in his *Breast Cancer Prevention Diet* says to cut out sugars. This is most important to prevent getting a second cancer.

Fight cancer before it starts with good eating practices

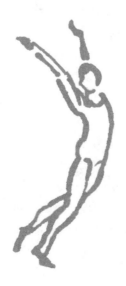

Natural Cholesterol In Your Diet

Cholesterol has gotten a bum rap from the media and manufacturers of many packaged foods. Advertising copy on packages promotes sales by saying that a product has no cholesterol. Cholesterol is not a villain to be booed and shunned.

Your body needs cholesterol for several functions

First, cholesterol is in the structure of the membranes of every cell in your body and in your brain. Second, it is the basic molecule that after minor modification can be changed into vitamin D, sex hormones or adrenal-cortical hormones. Third, as a component of bile acids it acts like a detergent to help break dietary fat into smaller globules so pancreatic lipase can start to digest them and they can be absorbed from the small intestine as chylomicrons (oils with a thin layer of protein and cholesterol molecules).

When you eat less cholesterol, your liver must make more of this vital chemical

A normal adult excretes 1,100 mg. of cholesterol a day. About 250 mg. of this is from the typical American diet and 850 mg. is made by the liver. Dietary cholesterol forms part of the fat globules absorbed from the intestine. Some goes to the liver where it can be changed to bile and ultimately excreted in the feces.

Low-density-lipid (LDL)-cholesterol is made by the liver from active-acetate, the end product from any carbohydrate, protein or fat. Molecules are called low density because they are light, with 50 percent cholesterol and 50 percent fat. LDL cholesterol is damaging to your cardiovascular system *only if it is in excess and isn't used normally.* The Doctors Eades say that certain very small molecules of LDL cholesterol are more dangerous than larger molecules of LDL cholesterol. These smaller molecules can get into the lining of blood vessels to start plaque.

In order to be carried in the blood, all fat-cholesterol globules have protein molecules attached. Lipoprotein (a) is a specific protein attached to some low-density cholesterol lipids. As a _marker,_ it correlates well with the danger that a particular kind of LDL cholesterol and fat might be deposited in or on vessel walls. However lipoprotein (a) itself doesn't cause this deposit.

You need both LDL and HDL cholesterol

The term "bad cholesterol" is misleading. Only when the ratio of LDL cholesterol is more than three times that of HDL cholesterol is there a problem. The LDL cholesterol is carried by the blood along with HDL cholesterol to the glands that use it to make adrenal steroids or sex hormones. The HDL (high-density-lipid) cholesterol molecules are heavier because they contain only 20 percent cholesterol with fat plus protein and phosphorus. HDL and LDL cholesterol interact together to make cell membranes. Some HDL goes back to the liver to make bile salts and be excreted. Some cholesterol attaches to fiber in the diet. Intestinal bacteria can metabolize the rest of it before excretion. HDL can be raised by eating more protein and fat or by vigorous exercise. The triglyceride (fat) level in the blood should be no higher than HDL cholesterol for good health.

A diet high in manufactured fructose raises LDL cholesterol to an unhealthy high level

Fructose in the diet raises the cholesterol of both types of diabetics and even non-diabetics. As mentioned earlier, a study by Dr. John Bantle of men on high fat diets showed that those who got carbohydrate calories as simple starch showed no change in blood cholesterol or lipids. Others on the same high fat diet who got the same 20 percent of their carbohydrate calories as fructose showed an increase in both cholesterol and blood fats. Moreover, 10 of the men who already had high insulin levels had a 30 percent average increase of cholesterol and 50 percent increase of triglycerides (fats). The liver transforms fructose into fat and the worst very-low-density cholesterol which can be deposited inside the lining of blood vessels as well as going into fat cells. The next chapter shows that a manufactured fat known as *trans fat* also raises LDL cholesterol.

Some people have very high total cholesterol because they inherited defective genes

About one person in a million gets a bad gene from both his parents. His cholesterol can be from 650 to 1000 mg. per 100 ml. of blood. One in 500 people has a single faulty gene with cholesterol in the 250 to 550 range. In both cases, they have an increased chance of a heart attack before age forty. Over the years, doctors have tried to lower the cholesterol of these patients with various methods, including clearing it from the intestine or the blood and blocking its synthesis. Many of these helped a little or had negative side effects.

The vitamin niacin (nicotinic acid) in large doses has lowered cholesterol by 40 points or more. Niacin dilates small blood vessels. Most patients didn't like the side effects, an itchy flush and sometimes heartburn and diarrhea, so niacin isn't used much. Robert Kowalski in *The 8-Week Cholesterol Cure* says that Enduracin, a sustained-release form of niacin, can reduce the level of the "bad" LDL cholesterol without the annoying flush of high levels of niacin. It should be monitored by your doctor and avoided by patients with previous liver damage.

Drugs called "statins" inhibit the production of cholesterol early in its synthesis in the liver. These are effective but should be used only by the people with the hereditary enzyme defect. Anyone else taking statin type drugs can be playing with fire. Since these drugs block the production of cholesterol, taking them ignores all the necessary actions of cholesterol. Your body always needs new cell membranes and a continual supply of adrenal and sex hormones. Even the manufacturers of some of these statins warn of possible liver or kidney damage or destruction of muscle cells. In fact the statin called Baycol was taken off the market because of this damage. Still, pharmaceutical companies have induced doctors to prescribe millions of dollars worth of other statins to fearful patients who think cholesterol causes heart attacks. Some drug companies imply that many more millions of people need them according to a new definition of high cholesterol. It makes more sense to cut out sugars, especially fructose, so the liver doesn't make excess cholesterol and fat from them.

In otherwise normal people, cholesterol values have been measured between 130 and 260. I remember in the 1950s and 1960s when patients with evidence of hypothyroidism were first given cholesterol tests before the more expensive thyroid tests. A high cholesterol level decreased after the thyroid deficiency was corrected. Other patients had high cholesterol values because of diabetes. Excess blood cholesterol is not automatically deposited in your blood vessels. As explained in the chapter on factors in cardiovascular disease, anything that damages the lining of blood vessels can cause a deposit of cholesterol. This includes nicotine, high insulin, high fructose, homocysteine, *Chlamydia pneumoniae* bacteria and high blood pressure. Since the body makes more cholesterol than is taken in with the diet, look to lifestyle changes if you want to lower your blood cholesterol.

Drug manufacturers make you think that the lower your blood cholesterol, the better. This is not true. Doctors Michael and Mary Eades have a diagram in *The Protein Power Life Plan* that incorporates the results of many studies (this chart is repoduced on the next page, with their permission). It shows a healthy middle range of cholesterol between 110 and 250 mg per 100 ml. blood. Even though deaths from cardiovascular disease rose with levels over 280, deaths from all causes rose dramatically with levels below 100. These included cancer, suicides and accidents. The

Doctors Eades say that two well-controlled studies in Finland showed more deaths in men who were taking cholesterol-lowering drugs than in controls. They say the famous Framingham study has failed to show a clear cause-and-effect relationship

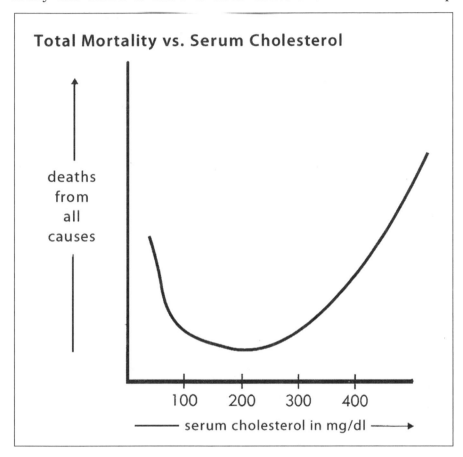

between cholesterol levels and heart disease.

For more than 10 years, the Drs. Eades have lowered their patients' cholesterol without drugs by using a diet containing adequate protein, good fats, low carbohydrates, special vitamins and natural antioxidants. They treated the cause of high cholesterol levels, usually too much sugar that produced too much insulin. Their patients' elevated cholesterol disappeared along with their obesity and type II diabetes.

Even so-called high cholesterol levels might not be dangerous. One athletic friend now in his sixties told me his cholesterol has never been below 240 and has tested at 270. He is very active and healthy. He has had little control of his diet because of living in deserts of the Middle East, jungles of South East Asia and elsewhere away from civilization. He doesn't take medications even though both his cholesterol and his blood pressure are considered above normal. He has never had a heart attack or related symptoms. A slender Asian woman told me her cholesterol was 239. Even though she had no cardiac symptoms, her doctor said that was too high and wanted to prescribe a statin drug. She decided to go on daily walks instead to increase "good" HDL cholesterol.

Don't get fixated by cholesterol levels. Elevated blood cholesterol is not from cholesterol in your food. It can be a sign that something else is wrong with your diet or individual physiology. Exercise and a natural diet higher in protein and fat can normalize your cholesterol. Nicotine and continued elevated blood insulin are probably most responsible for injuries in blood vessels that cause the deposit of cholesterol. A change in lifestyle can remove these causes without drugs or surgery. Most people should avoid expensive dangerous statin pills that interfere with the normal metabolism of cholesterol.

Your body needs and uses cholesterol

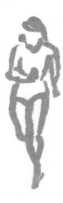

Trans Fats Are The Dangerous Dietary Fats

Artificially saturated fats, not naturally
saturated fats, are the ones to avoid.

Despite some of the advice of the past 30 years, you do not need to avoid naturally saturated fats. Human body chemistry has developed to use foods with saturated plant and animal fats as well as the unsaturated fats (those with one or more double bonds). Saturated fats have no double bonds to combine with oxygen, so they are less reactive both outside and inside the body. Chinese restaurant owners often cook with lard, a natural saturated fat, since it doesn't go rancid easily. Oleomargarine, an artificially saturated fat, is once again considered inferior and less healthy than butter, because of its unnatural manufactured fats, known as *trans* fats.

Trans fats are artificially saturated and should be avoided

In 1910, scientists started turning oils into solid fats by heating them to temperatures from 250 to 400 degrees Fahrenheit with hydrogen under pressure in the presence of a nickel catalyst. They knew that oils are liquid at room temperature because the double bonds they contain allow the molecules to be curved and slide over one another. Solid fat has straight chains of fatty acids with hydrogen atoms fastened on *all* the carbons so they can stack close to one another in a compact form. Until recently, scientists were unaware that *how* the extra hydrogen atoms were fastened affected the body's use of the resultant fats.

In natural solid fats like dairy butter or coconut butter, the added hydrogen atoms extend in the same direction and are called *cis* fats. Half of the hydrogen in the artificially hydrogenated fats extend in the opposite direction, making them *trans* fats. These became the solid fats known for over 90 years as Crisco shortening or oleomargarines. Since they don't get rancid as quickly as the oils from which they are made, they have been used in manufactured foods for many years. Rancid fats and oils are dangerous because of the lipid peroxides formed. Peroxides can act as free radicals and disturb reactions within the cells.

Artificially hydrogenated fats react differently in the body than do natural saturated fats

Trans fats don't interact with intracellular enzymes in the same way cis-fats do. When trans fats are incorporated into cell membranes, they make them stiffer. Stiff cell walls in blood vessels make them prone to injury. Trans fats are the ones most likely to be deposited in your blood vessels as plaque. Therefore, trans fats are one of the causes of cardiovascular disease. They also have a negative effect on aging because they make cell walls less flexible in all parts of the body.

Dr. Mary Enig, a respected researcher at the University of Maryland, has been studying the effects of trans fats since the 1970s. Her results ran counter to the medical establishment, which had blamed animal fat for cardiovascular disease and urged people to eat margarine instead of butter. She knew she posed a threat to the billion-dollar food oil industry. Hydrogenated fats made from corn oil or cottonseed oil are much cheaper than other fats used in manufacturing. The resulting bakery goods have a very long shelf life.

Enig's book, *Know Your Fats: The Complete Primer for Understanding Fats, Oils, and Cholesterol*, has analyzed other scientists' research on trans fats, in both humans and other animals. She lists other effects in addition to the stiffening of cell membranes and the tendency to be deposited as plaque in blood vessels. Trans fats can raise the total cholesterol by 20-30 mg. per 100 ml. of blood. This occurs by raising LDL ("bad") cholesterol while lowering HDL ("good") cholesterol. The more trans fats consumed, the greater this cholesterol effect.

Trans fats also raise lipoprotein (a), the marker chemical for an increased risk of heart attack. At the same time, these fats alter the insulin response to glucose and increase the potential for diabetes. Dr. Enig also reports negative effects related to sex. Males eating a lot of trans fats have lower testosterone levels and more abnormal sperm. Females can have offspring with lower birth weight. In both lactating humans and other mammals, there is less total fat in their milk. This interferes with the normal growth of infants. Trans fats can cause other biochemical and physiological abnormalities. Research by other investigators has shown that these fats contribute to cancer, diabetes, and abnormal immune responses.

Foods containing trans fats have a long shelf life

This is good for producers, distributors and grocers, but not good for your health. Advertisers brag about foods low in cholesterol and saturated fat. They seemed to ignore the possibility that trans fats might be one of the causes of the increase in many metabolic diseases. In 2002, the Food and Drug Administration took notice of the research on trans fats. It now suggests that labels on food products list the percentage of trans fats as well as that of saturated fat. If you don't see it on a label, avoid any food that lists even a partially hydrogenated vegetable oil. It contains trans fats. Don't be fooled if packages or containers list an oil, then a partially hydrogenated version of the same oil. Trans fats have always been partially hydrogenated. The manufacturers add only enough hydrogen to make the resultant fat solid at room temperature. Junk food with trans fats is truly junk.

Since 1950, and especially after 1980, other oils besides cottonseed and corn oil have been used to make margarine. Margarine made from safflower, canola and other poly-unsaturated oils came to market at higher prices more recently. A soft margarine is somewhat better than a hard one, but no amount of trans fat is as healthy as a natural solid fat like butter or organic lard or suet.

Not all plant oils are nutritious

Avoid anything with cottonseed oil. It can contain traces of the many insecticides used on cotton plants. Olive oil is one of the best oils to use both for salads and in cooking. With only one reactive double bond, it is solid in the refrigerator but liquid at room temperature. Olive oil is not as likely to be oxidized into peroxides as are most poly-unsaturated vegetable oils. Most of these oils contain an abundance of linoleic acid. This omega-6 fatty acid is already too high in most modern diets, mainly in salad dressings and baked goods.

A later chapter will explain how three essential fatty acids help your body's immune system respond to stress. This happens when there is a good ratio of the linolenic omega-3 acids to the linoleic omega-6 fatty acids. (1:4 instead of the 1:20 in the average diet.) Good sources of omega-3 acids are fish oils, flax oil and walnuts. Soy oil has both omega-3 and omega-6 fatty acids. Other nuts and seeds have mostly omega-6 fatty acids. Nuts with either type of poly-unsaturated essential fatty acid are prone to get rancid so should be kept in the refrigerator.

The taste of a rancid oil or nut warns you it is not as healthy as when fresh. Trans fats, being non-reactive, don't taste different. You don't realize that you shouldn't eat them. I remember some vanilla wafers I was going to use in a special dessert one Christmas. I ate a couple but plans changed so they stayed on the shelf. A year later, I could have used them because even in the opened box, they still tasted fine. The trans fats were so non-reactive, the cookies had not changed. A long shelf life is not a virtue.

Trans fats are dangerous fats
they are the ones you should avoid

Factors in Cardiovascular Disease

The idea that dietary saturated fat and cholesterol produce heart disease seems to be ingrained in the national psyche.

Recently, two writers of separate short stories won prizes using this premise. Their quite different stories told of disgruntled wives who intentionally killed their husbands in less than two years by feeding them rich, fatty, cholesterol-laden food. The deaths were considered natural and the wives lived happily on the husbands' insurance. This is pure fiction. It won't work.

Does saturated fat and cholesterol in the diet cause cardiovascular disease?

The origin of fatty plaque might not be obvious. Doctors who see fatty plaque in diseased blood vessels are convinced it must have come from eating food containing lots of saturated fat and cholesterol. They tell their patients the plaque was caused by too many hamburgers and french fries. They say not to eat egg yolks, butter or other saturated fat. Yet on a supposedly heart-healthy diet, the patient has to come back in months or years for another operation because of clogged arteries.

Other items in the diet that might cause fatty plaque are ignored by the doctors. The liver makes cholesterol and fat from carbohydrates in the diet. Consuming sugars has increased in the last 100 years from a few pounds to more than 150 pounds per person per year. Meanwhile, eating animal fat has gone down. Inappropriate information seized on by doctors and the media was based on animal studies. Rabbits fed cholesterol did deposit it in their blood vessels. However, they are herbivores, so cholesterol is foreign to them. In another study, saturated fat fed to monkeys caused plaque in their arteries. Monkeys are vegetarians, so they wouldn't use this fat normally as do chimpanzees and humans, both omnivores.

Let's look at it from an evolutionary standpoint. If fat is so bad for the coronary arteries of the heart, why do lymph vessels from the small intestine collect globules containing fat and carry them up the thoracic duct to the main vein that goes directly to the heart? It is because the heart muscle prefers to burn fat, since it's more efficient than glucose for a muscle that is working continually. Man and his Paleolithic ancestors have been eating eggs and fatty meat for millennia without heart disease.

What is the mechanism of cardiovascular disease?

In 1972, Canadian doctors Wilfred and Evan Shute published *Vitamin E for Healthy and Ailing Hearts* to show this vitamin's action in preventing heart disease. If there's not enough vitamin E, the doctors contended, some cholesterol in the blood is changed by peroxides and sticks to the walls of coronary vessels. This is then engulfed by certain white blood cells to form plaque. More collects until a person has a heart attack. The Shutes showed that vitamin E protected 30,000 high-risk patients from heart attacks. However, in the next decade, instead of trying vitamin E, North American doctors performed 200,000 coronary bypass operations. They replaced damaged vessels instead of preventing the damage.

Some people think of cardiovascular disease as the decrease of blood flow to heart muscle because of fat and cholesterol collecting inside blood vessels, like mineral deposits in a water pipe. This is too simplistic, according to P. Libby in "Atherosclerosis, a New View" in the May, 2002 issue of *Scientific American*. Simple plaque causes the vessel to expand outward so blood can flow normally. Libby says a microscopic analysis of atherosclerotic arteries showed that most fat and cholesterol does not adhere to the inside but is deposited within the tissue of vessel walls. When the smallest LDL cholesterol molecules pass through the lining of the walls, they can combine with oxygen, free-radicals or glucose. This attracts macrophages, T-cells and other white cells, causing inflammation. Macrophages engulf LDL molecules and become fat-filled foam cells, eventually covered by a layer of fibrin or calcium. If this layer is weakened by high blood pressure, by chemicals such as nicotine or high insulin or certain viruses or bacteria such as *Chlamydia pneumoniae*, blood clots form at the area of injury. A dislodged clot can cause a heart attack.

The medical establishment still puts major blame on saturated fat and cholesterol for heart disease, ignoring an International Atherosclerosis Project, reported by investigator, L. A. Solberg in a Jan. 22, 1970, Norwegian medical journal. It showed, by way of 31,000 autopsies in 15 countries, that no correlation exists between animal-fat intake and serum cholesterol level or the amount deposited in arteries. The 50-year Framingham Study, begun in 1948, has been misinterpreted by many in the medical establishment. Dr. William Costelli, director of the study, reported in a 1992 article in *The Archives of Internal Medicine* that the people who ate the most calories, most saturated fat and the most cholesterol were the leanest and the most physically active. However, Costelli's conclusions here and in other writings still advocate not eating saturated fat. In America, the amount of animal fat eaten has gradually declined since 1920. Meanwhile, cardiovascular disease has increased. It is now the biggest killer of both men and women over 65.

Much heart disease is due to years of smoking

Nicotine causes small blood vessels to clamp down just as it causes the heart to pump faster and raise blood pressure. Small vessels in the heart can be injured. If the arteries to the heart have been made smaller, it's an invitation to a heart attack. The realization that smoking is the leading cause of heart disease came several years after the correlation of smoking with lung cancer. Many smokers who get no exercise, eat faulty diets and have a lot of stress do indeed suffer heart attacks. Their doctors then perform surgery to bypass their clogged coronary arteries. In cases of less severe chest pain and only partially blocked vessels, the doctor inserts a catheter with a balloon up the vessels to the heart and flattens out the fatty plaque. Doctors and patients alike think because the plaque contains fat and cholesterol, it must have come from those substances in the patient's food. The patient stops smoking and cuts out fat and cholesterol from his diet. However, he may again have cardiac symptoms years or even months later.

The role of sugars in causing heart disease

Besides smoking, a modern diet high in sugar and low in fiber contributes to cardiovascular disease as shown separately by Dr. Sanford Siegal, Dr. Diana Schwarzbein and others. Innumerable studies have shown that when primitive peoples adopted modern Western diets, they were no longer as metabolically healthy. They developed diabetes, heart disease, kidney disease and cancer. Among others, Dr. Siegal said the lack of dietary fiber was the major cause of metabolic diseases.

Factors that affect the results of heart disease studies

The majority of the medical establishment continued to blame meat and dietary fat.They chose to ignore observations showing that the diets of most urban, formerly primitive people are now loaded with sugar in nutritionally empty soft drinks or packaged high carbohydrate foods. The fact that Arctic peoples didn't suffer from heart disease on their former high-protein, high-fat diet was dismissed because they were protected by eating fish oils. Did no one consider that when they lived in town they might still be getting these from eating salmon but their bodies were overwhelmed by the high sugar junk food and soft drinks they were now using? These are the items in a Western diet that can cause diabetes and heart disease.

The majority opinion also discounted the fact that Mongolian herdsmen don't suffer cardiac disease despite their diet of mare's milk, yogurt, hard curds and meat. African herdsmen also have consumed a high-protein diet for centuries. It included blood from their cattle along with milk but not much fiber. Therefore, fiber is only one of the reasons some primitive diets are superior to modern ones. The primitive people who eat lots of meat and/or dairy products stay healthy until they start two harmful habits that come with civilization: smoking and drinking sugary soft drinks. These are the habits most responsible for heart disease and diabetes in a modern lifestyle.

Middle-aged Australian aborigines from the city suffering from diabetes were studied by Dr. Kerin O'Dea, Health Research Director, Darwin, Australia. They were paid to spend seven weeks back in the bush as hunter-gatherers on their native diets. They ate mainly animal foods that included insects and snails as well as some kangaroo meat. The diet had high-protein, moderate fat and low carbohydrate. Results were amazing. Blood glucose and blood insulin both dropped by almost half to near normal values. Triglycerides, or blood fats, fell by a factor of three to a normal value. These changes occurred despite the fact the people got less exercise in the bush than in the city. Without an incentive to stay in the wild, they returned to the city and the ease and taste of a Western diet.

Fructose raises levels of LDL cholesterol

As mentioned in the chapter on insulin, John Bantle, M.D. gave fructose to diabetics to prevent spikes in insulin caused by glucose. It worked in both type I and type II diabetics, but their cholesterol increased, especially the low-density "bad" cholesterol. Fructose also raised the cholesterol of non-diabetics. Sheldon Reiser, PhD at a U.S. Department of Agriculture research center studied two groups of men both eating high fat diets. Those who consumed simple starch [readily made into glucose] showed no change in blood cholesterol or lipids. Others on the same high fat diet who got 20 percent fructose had an increase in both cholesterol and blood fats. Moreover, 10 of the men who had previous high insulin levels had a 30 percent average increase in cholesterol and 50 percent increase in triglycerides (fats). Their livers had changed the fructose into fats and LDL cholesterol. Remember, besides being deposited into fat cells, these substances in the blood stream can get into the lining of blood vessels to repair injuries and become plaque.

High levels of fructose cause other problems

Fructose promotes the abnormal clotting of blood; clots sticking to vessel walls can cause plaque to form. Fructose directly damages the lining of blood vessels even more than the high levels of insulin caused by too much sugar. High fructose also interferes with the absorption of copper, a mineral that promotes several cellular reactions including making red blood cells. Fructose can increase the number of free radicals in the body. It also causes the cross-linking of proteins making tissues less flexible. This is a factor in aging of the skin and other parts of the body.

Fructose is worse than sucrose (table sugar) because in addition to harming your blood vessels it causes the liver to produce LDL cholesterol and other blood lipids and get them into your blood stream. The high-fructose corn syrup in a big soft drink can damage your arteries and cause the clots and fatty plaque of cardiovascular disease. A high-sugar beverage is much more dangerous to your heart than a hamburger from a grass-fed steer (not one from a factory farm).

Homocysteine can show a risk of heart disease better than levels of LDL cholesterol and blood fats

Some people with slightly elevated cholesterol values have had heart attacks. Attempts to lower their blood cholesterol by diet or drugs have no effect. These patients have a metabolic defect related to the homocysteine in their blood. Homocysteine is a simple amino acid on the pathway between two other amino acids, methionine and cysteine. More than 30 years ago, Dr. Kilmer McCully published a theory that high homocysteine levels can predict the possibility of a heart attack. But at that time, the medical community was concentrating on cholesterol.

Patricia Fallest-Strobl, David Koch and others at the University of Wisconsin Medical School have recently published an article titled "Homocysteine: A New Risk Factor for Atherosclerosis." They point out that 15 percent of patients with premature heart attacks had high levels of homocysteine instead of high levels of cholesterol and other lipoproteins. One of their patients, whose father died of a heart attack at age 46, had a normal blood sugar, slightly high total cholesterol of 236 and an HDL of 88, showing plenty of good high-density cholesterol. However, his homocysteine was almost two-and-a-half times normal. The doctors prevented a potential heart attack by giving him multivitamins with extra folic acid.

A high blood level of homocysteine can be caused by a genetic absence of the enzyme that helps in its metabolism. It can also be associated with chronic diseases like hypothyroidism, kidney failure, psoriasis and some cancers. Most often it occurs because of a dietary deficiency of folic acid, vitamins B6 and B12. Folic acid is found in leafy green vegetables. Yeast and liver are good sources of Vitamin B6 (pyridoxine). Vitamin B12 is dependent on animal products in the diet. Many elderly people don't get enough of all three in their food, but can take them in pill form. One doctor advises his patients to take betaine (trimethylglycine) as well, to help change homocysteine into methionine.

Now more doctors are testing for homocysteine. A level greater than 12 micromoles is high. This is treated with diet, vitamins and amino acid therapy without the side effects or dangers of cholesterol-lowering statin drugs.

C-reactive protein can be another sign of an increased risk of heart disease

This special protein has been known for years to increase along with inflammation anywhere within the body. Various white blood cells increase during this process. They are helpful when they engulf or destroy bacteria or viruses, but they can also accumulate around the plaque that is patching damage in the lining of blood vessels. A high level of C-reactive protein in the blood indicates that the plaque is easily dislodged. Plaque or a resultant blood clot might be carried into a small coronary blood vessel to cause a heart attack.

Patients who get angina (heart pain) not relieved by nitroglycerine or other medication are the ones with the highest levels of C-reactive protein. This predicts a possible heart attack better than the level of blood cholesterol and fats. It is even more important than how much the vessels were made smaller by the accumulation of fatty deposits.

Many studies challenge the simplistic avoidance of cholesterol and saturated fat

These are reviewed by Janeen Hunt, Data analyst/ researcher at Immutopics, a research and development laboratory in San Clemente, California, in an article with extensive references. It is reproduced with Hunt's consent in the addendum to this book. Janeen Hunt has analyzed the literature on the relationship of diet, fat and cholesterol. Her annotated bibliography shows in 25 points that total cholesterol is not a strong indicator of the risk of cardiovascular disease. Even the relation of fat to total cholesterol is ambiguous. In fact, low fat diets decrease "good" HDL cholesterol. Dietary cholesterol doesn't increase total blood cholesterol but permits the liver to make less of it from carbohydrates. Hunt concludes, "Therefore, fat in the diet has never been the problem. Avoiding fat is the problem."

Endocrinologists Dr Richard Bernstein and Dr. Diana Schwarzbein would agree. They find that cutting carbohydrates and ignoring the fat produces improvement in heart disease, diabetes and obesity. In *The 8-week Cholesterol Cure,* Robert Kowalski states that a diet low in saturated fat and cholesterol lowered his cholesterol an insignificant 7 percent. His use of oat bran and a type of niacin produced a much lower level. But as mentioned earlier, other factors are predict heart attacks better than cholesterol level.

The fact that 35% of the men in the Framingham study with cholesterol levels between 150 and 200 had heart attacks should have caused Dr. Costelli and his cohorts to look at other factors besides cholesterol levels. It should not make anyone try to lower his cholesterol below 150 as some have suggested. As mentioned earlier, smoking, a low-fiber, high-sugar diet, high homocysteine levels or inflammation as indicated by C-reactive protein are better predictors of heart disease.

The Harvard Nurses' Health Study, starting in 1976 of more than 84,000 nurses, reported by Dr. Frank Hu and other Harvard medical researchers, showed that nurses who ate the most fish or took omega-3 fatty acids in capsules during a 16-year period had the least cardiovascular disease. Linolenic acid is the essential omega-3 fatty acid found in flax oil and walnuts as well as in the fat of cold water fish. This confirms foreign studies that men who ate an ounce or more of fish daily had a 40 to 50 percent decrease in deaths from heart disease. Eating fish correlates better in keeping the heart healthy than how much fiber, red meat or trans fats (margarine) people eat. It also is more important than the ratio of animal fat to polyunsaturated oils or if subjects took aspirin.

Alternatives to anti-cholesterol drugs

You have probably seen extensive advertisements on network television and magazines like the AARP bulletin that make you think you should take an anti-cholesterol drug. They imply that if you don't smoke, are exercising and eating a "heart-healthy" diet with no saturated fat and no eggs but still have high cholesterol, you need an anti-cholesterol drug. Some say half of all Americans need these statin drugs. Before trying these potentially dangerous drugs that interfere with the liver's ability to make cholesterol, it makes more sense to try a *different diet,* one that provides more fiber, folic acid and vitamins. The diet should cut out sugars, especially high-fructose corn syrup. It should have butter but no margarine or bakery goods with trans fats. It should allow cholesterol and some natural saturated fat along with adequate proteins and essential fatty acids.

The medical establishment and the media still say that a heart-healthy diet is low in fat and cholesterol. Pritikin said to avoid even the fat in plant foods like avocados. Most seem to disregard the carbohydrates and manufactured foods a person is eating. Look at pamphlets from your HMO or those found in senior centers to verify the emphasis on a low-fat diet.

Some doctors believe that you might not need surgery to deal with plaque in coronary arteries

In *The Best Alternative Medicine,* Dr. Kenneth Pelletier describes a non-surgical program at Stanford University School of Medicine. It shows a 50 percent decrease in the need for heart surgery in the patients studied. The program includes lifestyle changes, but does rely on medication.

Dr. Dean Ornish's Program for Reversing Heart Disease has a more comprehensive protocol. His method includes relaxation techniques, yoga-based stress management and support groups plus exercise, a vegetarian diet and no smoking. After a year, Dr. Ornish, professor at the University of California, San Francisco, who heads a clinic in Sausalito, claims his patients cleared their arteries of plaque so they didn't need surgery. Mutual of Omaha was the first company to announce it would pay the $5,000 cost of Dr. Ornish's program. Other insurance companies soon realized this extensive program is more cost-effective than surgery of any kind. By tackling major causes of heart disease, symptoms requiring surgical correction are prevented.

It seems clear the Ornish program can prevent future heart attacks and help clear partially clogged arteries. Patients should realize that the Ornish protocol emphasizes the factors of stress-reduction techniques, group support and adequate exercise. This non-surgical program takes time and dedication by the patient but might save his life. It keeps him away from an operating room.

Hospitals are becoming dangerous as bacteria become resistant to drugs. One friend had a successful coronary bypass operation but died a few days later because of a drug-resistant lung infection.

Dr. Ornish's stress reduction techniques might be more important than his strict vegetarian diet and avoidance of saturated fat and cholesterol. We need a well-publicized study using all of Dr. Ornish's lifestyle changes but with a diet including plenty of vegetables, moderate amounts of eggs and butter, small servings of good quality meat (organic, wild, grass-fed or from local small farms), but with no sugars or manufactured foods. I predict these patients would also show a reduction of arterial plaque and remove the necessity of any kind of cardiovascular surgery or the use of the potentially dangerous statin drugs that have harmed liver, kidneys or muscles in some patients.

Other prescription drugs only relieve symptoms but don't cure heart disease. Even if yoga, meditation, moderate exercise and meeting with a support group take a couple of hours a day, the cost is low compared to several surgeries or a fatal heart attack that could have been prevented.

If cardiac disease can be caught early, there is no need for surgery. It seems wasteful that some patients have had second coronary bypass surgeries to restore circulation to their hearts instead of trying other diets and stress reduction methods. No one would keep getting new engine tune-ups without first changing the dirty oil in his car. Similarly in the human body, no operation is more than a temporary fix if the underlying metabolic condition isn't changed. In certain people, correcting a homocysteine problem is as important in preventing cardiovascular disease as getting the proper balance of insulin and glucagon to prevent diabetes.

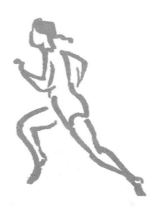

What you can do to lessen chances of a heart attack

- Stop smoking or never start. Nicotine raises blood pressure and causes blood vessels to clamp down which can injure the lining of your blood vessels.

- Avoid sugars. High glucose can cause high insulin that injures the lining of blood vessels. High fructose can produce injuries and cause the liver to make blood fats and low-density cholesterol. Both sugars can encourage fatty deposits in coronary arteries and other blood vessels. Both increase the possibility of blood clots.

- Avoid trans fats in margarine and many manufactured bakery goods.

- Take vitamin E to prevent deposits of oxidized LDL-cholesterol in your blood vessels..

- Get plenty of folic acid and vitamins B6 and B12 to avoid high homocysteine.

- Eat a diet high in vegetables for their fiber, vitamins and antioxidants.

- Do aerobic exercise to increase the efficiency of coronary vessels in the heart. Exercise also increases the HDL cholesterol in your blood, further helping your heart.

- Change your lifestyle to reduce stress. Try yoga and meditation to decrease your blood pressure and to eliminate the stress hormones that can injure blood vessels.

Succeeding chapters on stress, healthy diets and exercise will expand on these measures.

What Could Be More Harmful Than Obesity?

*Chemicals in body fat can be more harmful
than obesity itself. Obesity is a sign of defective
body physiology, not a cause of disease.*

It may precede or accompany diseases like diabetes, high blood pressure, atherosclerosis or cancer. However, a fat body itself isn't the culprit. Patients and doctors alike would do better to concentrate on the cause of the obesity. Besides not exercising enough, does the person eat a lot of manufactured foods with trans fats and high-fructose corn syrup? If a person eats meat, how is the animal raised?

Polynesian kings who got fat on yams, pork and coconut didn't have the metabolic diseases that some people say are caused by obesity. Coconut has been shunned by many people in the last 30 years because it contains a saturated fat. I saw the harm caused by this idea. On a vacation to Belize, I stayed at a comfortable but basic thatched-roof resort run by an American couple. They said that for several months when they were building it, they were low on grocery money. They ate a few of the coconuts from trees growing on their property, but stopped when they read that coconuts had saturated fat. Saturated fat was supposed to cause heart attacks. A local workman suggested that if they took up smoking, they wouldn't feel so hungry. Now as smokers, they're proud of being thin and think their calorie-restricted diet is healthy. As mentioned before, nicotine is one of the main causes of heart attacks, both by narrowing and injuring coronary blood vessels and increasing blood pressure. Being thin won't protect this couple's hearts from nicotine.

Does being thin promote health and prolong life?

Many people have the idea that getting very thin will give them a longer, healthier life. Some research on rats and other mammals suggests that they live longer if they take in 30 percent fewer calories. However, this data is not from the caloric intake of animals in the wild, but from those in laboratories. It makes sense to overfeed laboratory rats so they will grow faster, mature earlier and breed more rats for more experiments. Little mentioned is that the long-lived, calorie-restricted rats had a later sexual maturity. Food restriction delays puberty in most mammals. Perhaps this is the major reason for greater longevity when laboratory animals are fed less.

Are we giving our children too many calories? Is this one of the causes of early puberty and other problems? Some of our teenagers are too fat. Others start starving themselves and become too thin. As parents, we should be ensuring that children eat healthy, balanced diets, containing enough proteins and essential fats along with fruits, vegetables and whole-grains so they wouldn't be hungry for high-calorie fake foods that cause obesity and later metabolic disease. Young people should have some body fat, but morbid obesity is dangerous at any age.

Losing too much weight and being too thin can be unhealthy

Dr. David Lipscitz in his book, *Breaking the Rules of Aging,* says it is normal to gain weight as you move into middle age and beyond. This 10 percent or 15 percent weight gain then levels off. After age 70, the thinner you are, the more likely you are to die earlier than average. Lipscitz says in autopsies of the aged, there was no positive correlation between added weight and degree of atherosclerosis of arteries. In fact, many patients carrying extra pounds had healthier arteries than thin ones. Worst were those who lost weight, regained it and lost again several times throughout their lives. This raised their risk of death by 46 to 60 percent. These people often had increased total cholesterol but less "good"

HDL cholesterol.

Why should losing weight be so dangerous and cause a higher death rate in the thin elderly?

Is it because chemicals that had been sequestered in the fat came out into the blood stream? In the chapter on extreme diets, I say that pesticides given to animals, especially in the last weeks before slaughter when they are crowded together, concentrate in their fat. This is passed on to the humans who eat their meat, even if obvious fat has been removed. Anything that can act on the body chemistry of an insect to kill it is not healthy for the animal that absorbs it into its system. Steers have a short life, so there is no noticeable effect on the animal. Having been castrated, they don't produce sperm. However, people who eat the meat are gradually accumulating more and more pesticides in their body fat that can affect sex hormones and other body chemicals.

When this fat is mobilized and metabolized during a weight loss program, it can harm a person's brain and nervous system, the cardiovascular system, the liver and other organs. The faster the weight loss, the more toxins are released. The small amounts that were gradually accumulated did no apparent harm, but the massive load released from body fat in a crash diet could wreak havoc. Micro-injuries to the lining of blood vessels would be repaired by LDL cholesterol and fat, along with the toxins they contain. These stiffer, clogged arteries could cause high blood pressure, poor kidney function, heart attacks and even death.

Studies that seem to correlate meat with heart disease do not assess the presence of pesticides

As mentioned earlier, just because fat and cholesterol have been found in diseased arteries doesn't mean that these came from foods containing cholesterol and fat. The source of these substances is important in determining the effect on the body. Much of it was probably made from sugars. If any of it came from a deposit of dietary animal fat, it should have been analyzed. Is any of the material scraped from the arteries after an operation or autopsy routinely tested for pesticides? It doesn't make sense that meat, eggs and milk that humans have been eating for millennia without harm are now called the cause of heart attacks and other metabolic diseases.

Pesticides in dietary and body fat might have caused some of the diseases associated with obesity

The amount of pesticides used in American agriculture had increased tenfold in the 40 years since World War II, according to David Pimentel, professor of Agricultural Sciences at Cornell University. This continues to increase but is less effective as insects mutate. DDT, one of the most dangerous insecticides, had been banned in the U.S. since the early 1960s when it was shown to concentrate in human breast milk. (This didn't stop chemical companies from selling it to third world countries.)

Screening tests by the FDA on imported foods are quite ineffective, capable of detecting only 203 out of 400 pesticides. A General Accounting Office report in 1986, titled "Pesticides: Need to Enhance FDA's Ability to Protect the Public from Illegal Pesticides" also said that the FDA tests less than two-tenths of a percent of domestic produce. Even the level of risk from pesticides is based on an annual "average" diet of half a melon, one avocado, three cups of squash and similarly low amounts of other fruits and vegetables. We should be eating that much produce per week, not per year. Lesser amounts of pesticides come from vegetable sources, but you can't avoid them entirely by not eating animal fat. You would be better off by eating both produce and animal products from organic farms.

Obesity itself does not cause diabetes, heart disease and cancer

It's what you ate to get too fat that is ruining your health. It might have been sugar or high-fructose corn syrup in desserts or soft drinks. It might have been trans fats in margarine or packaged bakery goods or snack foods. It might have been the meat from animals raised in factory farms. Your goal should be to get healthy, not to just lose weight. Liposuction might remove fat, but if you continue to eat the same unhealthy foods, even in smaller quantities, you won't be healthy. Obesity is not a disease itself. It is only a sign of other potential diseases caused by a faulty diet and lack of exercise.

What You Can Do

Don't let yourself get fat from eating too much of any food, whether it contains fat, proteins or carbohydrates.

- Set a good example for your children by maintaining a medium weight. If you're now obese, never go on a crash diet.

- Lose weight slowly by increasing exercise and eating natural foods rather than manufactured food and drink.

- Forego liquid diet drinks that taste like milkshakes. They are a combination of chemicals that are not a good substitute for real food and often contain too few calories, slowing your metabolism.

- Buy local produce and organic meat and milk products or those from European countries to avoid adding more toxins to your body fat.

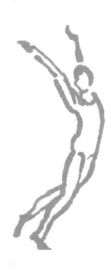

Stress, The Immune System & Essential Fatty Acids

The adrenals, small glands on top of the kidneys, produce hormones in response to stress.

Two types of stress hormones are from two different areas. The central part of the adrenal glands immediately releases adrenaline and nor-adrenaline into the blood stream. These cause a "flight or fight" reaction, increasing the heart rate and sending more blood to the lungs and muscles. These hormones don't last longer than the immediate crisis.

At the same time, other hormones are released from the outer part, the adrenal cortex. These are the long-term stress hormones known as the glucocorticoids. They can be produced for days or weeks, depending on circumstances.

Stress hormones are not bad *per se*, and are sometimes necessary. The body must be able to respond to physical stress and to defend against infections. But abnormal stress and its resulting chemical affects are damaging. Anxiety about a psychological or mental problem that seems out of a person's control can cause an increase of hormones from the adrenal cortex. Then the stress response is not appropriate and possibly damaging.

In 1936, Canadian scientist Hans Selye first described the stress response. He wrote articles and a definitive book in 1976. Since then, the layman has blamed stress for various physical and psychological ailments. Extensive research and many volumes have been written about the hormones of the adrenal cortex in the past 50 years. The link to intracellular chemicals that affect your immune system has been more recent.

About Adrenal Cortex Hormones

Cortisone was one of the earliest hormones studied that were made in the adrenal cortex. As reliable methods were discovered to test for it, a doctor noticed that when patients with rheumatoid arthritis got pregnant, their arthritis improved along with an increased level of cortisone in the blood. Later, doctors began giving cortisone for a variety of disorders related to the immune system. Unfortunately, there were side-effects with long-term use. It made some bacterial or fungal diseases worse. It often caused high-blood pressure, diabetes, osteoporosis and a change in fat distribution. A typical patient got a fat neck, puffy upper body fat and sometimes a buffalo hump.

Related glucocorticoids like prednisone seemed more benign but should also be used with caution. Ted started to use an inhaler containing one of the glucocorticoids to control the asthma he developed doing extensive driving through air polluted with automobile exhaust. A substance like pollen can become a true allergen when accompanied by an unrelated chemical. Either alone might not cause a reaction. Ted used the inhaler many times a day over the course of a year as his asthma got worse. His busy schedule didn't leave time to see his doctor to find out why it was getting harder to breathe. It was easier to ask for a refill of his prescription. A broken hip in this man, who was under 40, was his wake-up call. He had extreme osteoporosis with thin, fragile bones like some 80-year-olds. He had to have the hip joint replaced and probably will need surgery on the other hip. He now hobbles around like an old man. Corticoid use should be carefully monitored.

Hydro-cortisone rarely causes problems when applied to the skin to reduce the inflammation of minor rashes. Even this should not be continued if the rash persists. If it were caused by a fungus it might get worse.

DHEA, dehydro-epi-androstene-diol, is an adrenal hormone

more recently studied that has actions that oppose those of the cortisone type hormones. It is interesting that DHEA also reaches its highest levels in pregnancy. It acts on the connective tissue and muscles in the uterus. In fact doctors in Japan use extra DHEA to help the cervix to stretch for delivery of a baby. The normally high amounts of both cortisone and DHEA in pregnancy indicate that both are necessary for a healthy delivery.

All the chemicals made by the adrenal cortex have a basic structure of four interconnected rings, similar to that of cholesterol, from which they are made. The adrenal glands in both sexes also make both male and female sex hormones. (A man's testes make most of the testosterone and other androgens. A woman's ovaries make most of her estrogen and progesterone hormones.) The hormones made from DHEA in the adrenal glands can help keep muscles strong and maintain a normal fat distribution. If you buy DHEA pills, remember they must be accompanied by exercise to be effective for this. DHEA can also have positive actions on blood clotting and the immune system. However, it has the potential for abuse or side effects since it is the precursor for both male and female sex hormones. A woman might get facial hair. A man who takes high doses might get liver or kidney damage, similar to that of body builders who take too much testosterone. There must be a proper balance of cortisone and DHEA for health.

Other opposing chemicals made within the body cells affect immune responses

These include the eicosanoids and prostaglandins. Unlike hormones, they don't get into the blood stream but act within the cells that produce them. Three different eicosanoid series, with complementary functions, are all derived from the essential fatty acids in the diet. For good health, there should be a certain ratio of the fatty acids as described in the chapters on diets. These essential unsaturated fatty acids have double bonds between specific carbon atoms in the long chain. They are labeled omega-6 fatty acids or omega-3, indicating the carbon atom in the chain with the first double bond, starting from the acid end.

Series I eicosanoids are derived from linoleic acid, an omega-6 fatty acid, with two double bonds. They allow vessels and other body parts to react in normal non-stress actions, maintaining vessel size with minimal passage of liquid into the tissues.

Series II eicosanoids are from arachidonic acid, another omega-6 fatty acid, with four double bonds. These chemicals are released in stress situations and body injury, causing swelling, dilation of blood vessels, clotting and accumulation of white cells as needed. They help adrenal hormones and start repairing damage from wounds and microbial invaders. However, if you get too much linoleic acid, usually from polyunsaturated oils in your diet, it can be changed into too much arachidonic acid and contribute to allergic reactions.

Series III eicosanoids are from alpha linolenic acid, an omega-3 fatty acid with three double bonds. They act to modulate the action of the Series II chemicals. They protect against the excessive runaway activity of Series II on the joints, skin and lungs. For example, if Series III eicosanoids are deficient, Series II eicosanoids cause the lungs to try to repel common pollens as if they were dangerous bacterial invaders, one cause of an asthma attack. Series III also prevent the abnormal responses of auto-immune diseases like rheumatoid arthritis.

The body has developed needing all three types of eicosanoids. Problems occur when they're out of balance. Your body needs the essential fatty acids. Omega-3 fatty acids are important for your brain as well as your heart. Get the right proportions of all essential fatty acids from seeds, nuts, eggs, flax oil and fatty fish – as humans have been doing for centuries.

Don't be afraid of stress

Even if you can't control what sets off the stress response, you don't need to passively accept the damage the chemicals can do to your cardiovascular system, your brain and other organs. Work off the increased hormone levels by doing heavy physical labor or vigorous exercise as your ancestors did. The section on exercise will expand on this. You might forget the problem or figure out a solution.

Stress itself can be beneficial. Dr. Jeff Victoroff in *Saving Your Brain* says you need a moderate amount of stress. The stress of encountering a new situation or finding a solution to a problem can stimulate new cells in your brain. Stress keeps you feeling alive and able to tackle bigger challenges later.

Balance is the key to controlling the chemicals produced by stress. Your body has natural checks and balances. You can get into trouble by taking drugs that suppress the action of one of the opposing natural chemicals too much. If possible, avoid the conditions that produce the unwanted symptoms. Then you won't need the drugs to relieve them. Quiet meditation in addition to vigorous exercise can defuse the effects of chemicals released during stress. Take time for both to produce balance in your life.

Balance expresses the Golden Mean for better health.

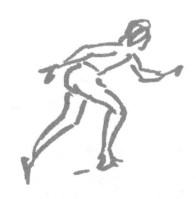

Allergies &
Food Addictions

*As mentioned in the chapter on stress, you need
a balance of body chemicals. Your body can
react to substances in the air and respond by
developing an allergy.*

Food can also cause allergies. Several authors show how specific foods are related to allergies. Some elements in food can
affect your brain as well as your body, leading to addictions in
some people.

A true allergy occurs when a substance acts as an antigen, a foreign invader

The antigen causes the body to produce large protein molecules
called antibodies that try to counteract it. Too often, there's an
overreaction, causing anything from a rash to asthma or even a
severe auto-immune disorder. A common antigen is the whey in
cows' milk. Other antigens include the gluten in wheat and other
grains. People allergic to peanuts can suffer asthma attacks just
from breathing air in a space where peanuts have been eaten.
Allergies causing hives, such as from eating strawberries, are
uncommon. Unfortunately, skin scratch tests for food allergies
are not as reliable as the skin tests for substances you breathe.
You might have to test for your own possible allergy or food intolerance.

Food sensitivity or intolerance is less severe than an allergy.
It causes bloating and gas or water retention in body tissues.
A common example is lactose intolerance, experienced by many
adults when they drink milk. Lactose or milk sugar occurs in

fresh milk. In fermented milk products like yogurt or cheese, the lactose has become lactic acid. Lactose sensitivity is an intolerance rather than an allergy because a small amount of lactose does not cause a problem. In fact, many placebo pills contain lactose (milk sugar).

Peter D'Adamo, in *Eat Right for Your Type*, says your blood type is related to food and body chemicals. His diagram shows the dispersal of humans from Africa across other continents. Blood type O is most common and started with early man, the prototype hunter-gatherer. When agriculture began in the Middle East, blood type A developed and people went north to Scandinavia. Blood type B people migrated across Asia and crossed the Bering Straits into American continents.

According to Dr. D'Adamo, just as people have antigens and antibodies in their blood that react with an incompatible blood type in a transfusion, they have antigens to certain chemicals in foods. He says the blood type O antigen is similar to the lectin, fucose. Blood type A antigen is similar to N-acetylgalactosamine. Type B antigen is like a d-galactose lectin. Eighty percent of the patients tested by the author [a select group] secrete these specific antigens in their saliva and other body fluids.

Eating according to blood type

This theory depends on the idea that food lectins (a sugar-protein complex) pass unchanged past intestinal cells into the blood stream. Blood types aren't the only genetic and biochemical differences between people. With a mixing of races over the centuries, only an isolated group would retain a single blood type or other distinctive characteristic. The write-up for blood type A didn't fit me or the optimal diet I got after years of experimenting. A friend who also has blood type A cut out meat, increased grains and felt more energetic, though she has gained weight. Why should types B and AB not eat chicken? An Asian friend says all of her family are type B and have no problem eating chicken.

It is possible that lectin intolerance might explain food sensitivities in some people. That everyone with a specific blood type should eat the same types of foods might be like believing that all those with the same astrologic sign have similar personalities.

A theory about grains

Doctors Michael and Mary Dan Eades have a different take on lectins. They say grains are foreign to a digestive system developed over many thousands of years in hunter-gatherers. They describe a "leaky gut" caused by a reaction to some chemicals in grains. Digestive products from too much grain can go through the small intestine unabsorbed and cause bacteria in the colon to multiply rapidly. These create gas, some bacteria move backward into the small intestine and form toxins that damage cell junctions and create leaks allowing whole molecules to get into the blood stream.

The Drs. Eades say a damaged small intestine can absorb partially digested lectins. These glyco-proteins often have amino-acid chains similar to those in certain body tissues. One wheat lectin is like that of joint cartilage. Some lectins in beans or other plants are similar to the covering of nerves or certain cells in the kidney or pancreas. In some people, this can cause auto-immune reactions where the body attacks itself as if repelling a foreign protein. This might explain maladies like rheumatoid arthritis, multiple sclerosis and ulcerative colitis. The Eades say that with a family history of any auto-immune disorder, stay away from most beans, wheat and corn. In fact they advise everyone not to eat too much of any grain product.

The Eades "leaky gut" theory might apply to certain people, but not most. A normal small intestine absorbs breakdown products of foods after enzymatic action. It is protected from harmful bacteria by tight junctions between cells in the duodenum where most digestion occurs and also in the jejunum where most absorption occurs in tiny projections as fine as velvet. These absorptive cells are renewed daily and the old cells are passed in the stools along with bacteria and fiber. In the ileum, the lower part of the small intestine, groups of white blood cells are just beneath the lining. These are ready to pounce on and engulf any bacteria either ingested with the food or backing up from a sluggish gassy colon. Most adults needn't worry about a leaky gut.

Babies can absorb large molecules from their undeveloped intestine

Many food allergies might have been unwittingly started by mothers who didn't have time to breast-feed and wanted to get their bottle-fed infants onto solid foods as soon as possible. All proteins weren't completely broken down into their component amino acids. The cellular lining of a baby's small intestine is still immature. Partially digested proteins might have passed through the lining of the small intestine into the blood stream to act as antigens. When the child later eats other foods that contain similar molecules, he might have an allergic reaction. This can be dangerous.

A friend told me that his daughter couldn't drink a cow's milk formula. Like a good many babies, she was switched to soy milk. Even later, she couldn't tolerate anything that contained whey, a common protein in cow's milk. Her mother read labels and rejected any food that had milk or whey as one of the ingredients. One day the child had a fig bar of a brand that had been okay in the past. She ended up in the hospital for a week because of a strong allergic reaction. The manufacturer had changed the recipe and included whey.

Eliminate a suspected food for several days or weeks to see if you feel better

One writer said that your pulse rate might increase several hours after eating a food that can cause allergies. If your heart rate increases and your old symptoms return when you try a small amount of that food, you might be allergic to it.

An allergy can produce a sudden reaction or one that occurs within two days. On the other hand, many people notice they have bloating or gas within a few hours or the next day after eating certain foods. This sensitivity is less dangerous than an allergy and is related to the amount consumed, as mentioned with lactose intolerance.

Harvey and Marilyn Diamond, authors of *Fit For Life*, suffered from many ailments that had begun when they were young. Some seemed related to foods they ate. They began a program they say helped them. While some aspects of the plan don't make sense and don't have a scientific basis, it has helped some people. The Diamond's diet plan says not to mix types of foods and to eat specific ones at a certain time of day; for instance nothing but fruit from the time of awakening until noon. In the afternoon and evening, eat lots of healthy vegetables, made tasty with genuine butter. They say not to eat meat or any manufactured food or beverages.

I think that since many people are sensitive to wheat, corn and milk, they would be healthier by not eating the typical breakfast of cereal and milk. Not eating snack foods high in grain products would also prevent effects of diet sensitivities.

An intolerance to a specific food often causes bloating and swelling

This is not a true allergy. Dr. Elson Haas in his book, *The False Fat Diet*, says food sensitivity can make you look 10 or 15 pounds heavier. He calls this "false fat" because it is mostly water. It can be lost quickly, unlike true fat that has to be burned for energy to disappear. Many restrictive low-calorie diets seem to give quick results. By not eating the foods that cause bloating, the person looks and feels thinner and sees a lower number on the scales. These people haven't lost any real fat and don't realize they only lost the "false fat" caused by their food sensitivity. They just moan that when they try to eat their usual food, it turns into fat by the next day. Water retention, not fat had made them weigh more again.

Wheat, sugar and dairy products cause many of these reactions: Haas lists eggs, corn, soy and peanuts as lesser sensitizers. He notes that diet soda and other common drinks can also cause bloating. I had such an experience a few years ago from orange juice. On a long cheap flight to Houston with plane changes, I had lots of orange juice. By the time I got to my hotel I noticed my belly was so bloated I couldn't fit into the long slim-waisted skirt I was going to wear to a formal wedding. I didn't have a heating pad so I tried a hot bath to decrease the bloating. Now I carry charcoal pills. They seem to absorb gas better than many over-the-counter pills. I don't remember such a problem before, but usually drink only small amounts of juice, preferring the whole fruit. Apparently, my body doesn't tolerate so much orange juice in one day, but it's not an allergy.

In a classic elimination diet, Dr. Haas' patients eat only the least reactive foods: apples, lamb, walnuts, salmon, lima beans and chard or kale. After a few days, they can add other foods one at a time. They should probably avoid grains, citrus, potatoes, tomatoes and shellfish even though these bother many fewer people than the seven foods listed earlier.

Dr. Haas classifies allergic food reactions according to the immuno-globulins (IgA, IgE or IgG) that are activated. If there isn't enough IgA in the intestinal lining, it is prone to leakage. IgE antibodies are involved in immediate allergic reactions, like the one mentioned earlier against whey. When IgG is stimulated, there is a delay of two to three days. Besides bloating, there can be flushing, hives, asthma, insulin resistance, diarrhea, migraine and rare conditions such as fibromyalgia.

Nitrites or nitrates in hot dogs or lunchmeat, sulfites in wine, Aspartame or the flavor-enhancer MSG can all combine with body cells and affect sensitive people directly, not by causing an allergy. Effects of any food reactions vary with the person.

You can avoid the foods that cause discomfort, but some people are like addicts

They crave the foods and continue to eat them despite feeling uncomfortable. Dr. Haas says that a reactive food depletes the serotonin in a person's brain. This causes a craving for that food along with sugars to increase brain endorphins. Low-blood glucose causes hunger; low serotonin can produce either anxiety or depression. You can feel tired because of low adrenalin. Any or all of the deficiencies make you like an alcoholic, craving the reactive food along with many carbohydrates. After finding out what causes the craving, Dr. Haas treats his patients with specific vitamins, the amino acid tryptophan, calcium and magnesium and one or two herbs, depending on the ailment. When patients feel healthy and energetic, they exercise and then lose regular fat. I think Haas has an excellent explanation of food sensitivities and using an elimination diet to see if intolerance to a certain food is causing false fat.

Another possible cause of bloating

Anne Louise Gittleman in *The Fat Flush Plan* has a different explanation. She says that the bloating that makes you feel fat is from food-related reactions to a toxic liver. Like other authors, she blames most sensitivities on dairy products, wheat and sugar. She also says that an overgrowth of intestinal yeast mimics food sensitivity causing discomfort and bloating. Gittleman says the liver is stressed by many factors, including low-fiber diets, sugars, trans fats, caffeine, chemicals, estrogen, anabolic steroids, anti-inflammatory drugs, anti-cholesterol drugs, anti-diabetic drugs and some herbal supplements. The toxic liver is alleged to cause high blood pressure, high cholesterol, fatigue, depression, rashes and cellulite as well as bloating and indigestion. Gittleman says to detoxify the liver with cranberry juice and a list of supplements, along with a high-protein diet.

I think the most good comes from staying away from the reactive foods. Protein helps since it contains essential amino acids mentioned by other authors. Similar to the effects reported by Dr. Haas, when bloating decreases, a person loses weight. However, I feel that any program that requires using a wide array of either herbs or drugs is best avoided. You might not know which item is causing side effects. *The Fat Flush* plan might work for some people but the underlying explanations don't seem verifiable. I wouldn't rush to flush.

Dr. Henry Chang in *Weight Lost Forever* tells his obese patients to weigh daily. A sudden weight increase should make them eat less the next day. I think the higher weight indicates false fat. Foods you are sensitive to would cause a noticeable sudden weight gain. It's avoiding these foods, not cutting total calories, that will keep you on track toward permanent weight loss and better health.

Brain chemicals can affect behavior

Though acetyl-choline is the most plentiful messenger chemical in the brain and the rest of the nervous system, other chemicals act within specialized structures in the brain. Endorphins are chemicals made in the body that act on the pleasure center of the brain. This center also responds to opiates and other drugs. I saw the power of this center when I considered doing graduate work in physiological psychology with Dr. J. Anthony Deutsch at the University of California in San Diego.

A rat's skull was partially removed so a thin electrode could be put into a specific part of the brain. The skull was replaced, with only a connector exposed. This could be wired to an apparatus where the rat could push a pedal to give a jolt of stimulation to his pleasure center. After a priming dose, rats kept stimulating that part of the brain, ignoring both food and an available sexual partner like true addicts. When disconnected from the apparatus, they behaved normally.

Endorphins may increase with addictive exercise or the good feelings that anorexics report as they get ever thinner. Other chemicals produced by certain cells in the brain affect behavior. These include serotonin, dopamine, nor-epinephrine and Gamma amino butyric acid (GABA). Addiction or problems such as anxiety, depression or extreme excitability occur when these chemicals are out of balance. Normal values exist in a wide range, probably genetically determined. Only extremes need correction.

Serotonin produces calmness and relieves anxiety. If dopamine is too low, a person is depressed. Nor-epinephrine makes a person energetic. If it's too high, he has a short fuse. GABA counteracts this in some people.

Julia Ross, author of *The Diet Cure*, says cravings and negative moods are from too little normal brain chemicals. As director of Recovery Systems in Marin County, California, she originally worked in a substance abuse clinic. She expanded her methods to the equally addictive reaction by some people to certain foods. In her book, she offers both a practical approach and a scientific explanation as to why some people can't lose weight no matter how hard they try. Ross says some foods, such as wheat and milk products, can be as addictive as caffeine, nicotine or illegal drugs. The worst addiction is to sugar and starches easily changed to sugar. Sugars increase endorphins and other chemicals in the brain. The person addicted to sugar continues overeating sweets to keep getting a sugar high. Even the artificial sweetener Aspartame, made by combining two amino acids, can be addictive. A person allergic or hypersensitive to certain foods will overeat them even when the symptoms aren't as pleasant as a sugar high - evidence of an addiction.

Brain chemicals can all be returned to normal by using specific amino acids

Ross' clinic recommends individual amino acids depending on the patients' blood tests, problems or emotional status. *The Diet Cure* is based on a 12-week plan. In all cases, cravings diminish the first week using the amino acids l-glutamine, 5-hydroxy tryptophan and d,l,-phenyl-alanine along with multivitamin, multimineral capsules as the person stays away from the addictive foods. Blood tests check for thyroid, adrenal or other problems. Ross says that glutamine, the only amino acid that the brain can metabolize like glucose, promotes normal brain function and removes the craving for sugars and even alcohol in many patients.

Ross also advises moderate exercise and relaxation techniques like meditation, warm baths, massages and soothing music. She advocates a high-calorie diet full of vegetables, fruits and oils as well as fish, whole eggs, meat or tofu. Specific suggestions as where to find supplements and holistic health practitioners as well as recipes make this a very practical book. By increasing certain brain chemicals, the patient is no longer addicted and can finally lose fat as well as feel more energetic. Patients use specific amino acids and other supplements for several weeks or months to straighten out their brain chemistry. They can then stop using the extra amino acids as they eat more protein in a lifelong diet to quench cravings for sweets, starches, stimulants and drugs. This plan might be the only way for the discouraged obese person to finally change his or her life and have a diet that works year-in and year-out.

Paul Rivas discusses four types of problems related to brain chemicals

In *Turn Off The Hunger Switch,* Rivas says that people with low nor-epinephrine (related to adrenaline) are constantly hungry. They keep eating, mainly starches. They feel tired all the time. Rivas says this is a common deficiency affecting mostly women. He calls these patients type N (nor-epinephrine deficient). The essential amino acid phenyl-alanine can increase nor-epinephrine. When nor-epinephrine is normal, a person feels energetic and doesn't need stimulants like caffeine, nicotine, sugar or various drugs.

Dopamine is a brain chemical related to depression

If it's too low, a person feels depressed. Dr. Rivas calls these patients type D. They often can't respond to sex and crave salty, fatty food as well as sweets. Julia Ross gives depressed patients tyrosine, since it can be changed into either nor-epinephrine or dopamine. Her patients feel energized and no longer need sweets, chocolate, stimulants or illegal drugs.

Serotonin is a brain chemical formed from the amino acid tryptophan

Serotonin promotes sleep when changed to melatonin. Adequate levels of serotonin prevent anxiety, irritability, PMS, phobias, low self-esteem and other negative feelings. Some of Ross' patients ate little all day, binged on carbohydrates at night, then threw up. These bulimic patients with their low-protein diets got no tryptophan in their food so they couldn't make serotonin or melatonin. Ross calls serotonin "our natural Prozac." Tryptophan or 5-hydroxy tryptophan can increase a depleted supply of serotonin. Patients then no longer need addicting foods or drugs. Dr. Rivas calls low serotonin patients Type S. They crave sweets, especially chocolate, and are obsessed with thoughts of food. They respond to stress by excessive eating. Some of Rivas' patients with low serotonin have a family history of alcoholism.

Rivas has different treatments for Types N, S, D, and C, the carbohydrate sensitive

The C patients can have any of the symptoms of the other types. They tend to eat mainly carbohydrates. They can't lose weight with low-calorie diets and moderate exercise. During their exercise, the carbohydrates they eat are used first so their bodies never need to metabolize their fat.

Rivas first starts all four types on the medicine Phentermine. He says it got an undeserved bad name when given with Fenfluramine. The cardiac problems of Phen-Fen were all caused by the Fenfluramine. Depending on the patient's type, Rivas gives other prescription drugs. If they object to drugs, his patients get specific amino acids plus herbal supplements containing ephedra and caffeine to increase metabolism. Type N patients get tyrosine to make norepinephrine. Types S, D, and C get 5-hydroxy tryptophan to stimulate serotonin. In addition, D and C types get the amino acid phenyl-alanine as well as SAMe (s-adenosyl l-methionine). This amino-acid compound must be taken with vitamin B6 or the methionine becomes homo-cysteine, implicated in cardiovascular disease.

Dr. Rivas says patients should continue with drugs or supplements even after reaching their ideal weight, though at half the dose. In addition, Type C people should avoid carbohydrates for the rest of their lives.

Drs. Rachael & Richard Heller wrote *The Carbohydrate Addicts Diet.* It was based on their personal experiences and that of their overweight patients since 1983. They define a carbohydrate addict as someone who focuses on food, never feels satisfied and gets tired in the middle of the afternoon. The person has extreme emotional ups and downs and can be angry or anxious for no apparent reason. All these symptoms come from too much insulin after eating carbohydrates. The Hellers say to eat two meals a day with protein, fiber and fat but no carbohydrates, then eat a daily reward meal from the four basic food groups.

There is no limit on amounts of foods, including carbohydrates and alcohol, as long as this meal takes no longer than one hour. They say that since insulin level wasn't raised during the day, only a moderate amount of insulin is made during the reward meal so blood sugar is back to normal in 60 minutes. It won't work if you eat even a little fruit in the no-carbohydrate meals. If non-carbohydrate addicts try the diet, their weight stays the same or increases with lavish reward meals. The Hellers' regimen might cause fat loss for the true carbohydrate addict who can stick to it day after day, year after year. However, eating "any amount of any food" during the reward meal might not make a person healthier despite being less fat. They still might develop other metabolic diseases.

Fixing sugar-carbohydrate addiction through diet

Dr. Diana Schwarzbein, in her book *The Schwarzbein Principle*, discusses the problems of sugar-carbohydrate addiction. She admits she was a sugar junkie while growing up. Now, as a clinical endocrinologist, she has cured many patients of carbohydrate cravings by altering their diets. Like other researchers, she says that many people keep trying to get the good feelings that come from eating sugars or starches because their brains are deficient in serotonin. Other substances, including caffeine, nicotine, chocolate, alcohol, cocaine, medicines like Phentermine, Ritalin, Prozac or Zoloft and herbs like Ma Huang, temporarily raise this pleasurable brain chemical. However, prescription drugs and stimulants make the problems worse. They aren't the way to raise serotonin.

Since most low serotonin is not genetic, it can respond to changes in diet, lifestyle and some hormones. Schwarzbein says to avoid all addicting substances, especially sugar. Continually trying to raise serotonin with carbohydrates leads to abnormally high insulin and finally insulin resistance. This causes most type II diabetes and much cardio-vascular disease. High-carbohydrate, low-protein diets don't have enough tryptophan. This amino acid is transformed in the body into serotonin, a calming, pleasurable brain chemical. Tryptophan can also become melatonin, the chemical that assures restful sleep.

Brain chemical levels exist in a wide range

Psychiatrist Dr. Michael Lesser, in *The Brain Chemistry Diet*, writes of deficiencies in certain brain chemicals after classifying his patients into six general types. Life experiences can modify a person's basic biochemistry. Only when a chemical is extremely high or low do any of these six types get into trouble.

Dr. Lesser also analyzes minerals like magnesium, copper and zinc. He prescribes vitamins, minerals, amino acids and supplements like St. John's wort and valerian in preference to prescription drugs. He says all types should exercise and eat five meals a day each with protein. These should be natural foods, not manufactured ones. All types should avoid sugar and caffeine. He says to take supplements depending on your type based on specific blood tests, not just his questionnaire.

Excess insulin after eating carbohydrates can affect a person's brain chemicals

People scoffed at the "Twinkie defense" used by Dan White after his shooting of politicians Harvey Milk and George Moscone in San Francisco in the late 1970s. However, many people who produce too much insulin in response to too much sugar are light-headed and emotionally unstable when blood glucose then gets too low.

Years ago, Dr. Benjamin Feingold said to change the diets of hyperactive children. He said to restrict sugar and keep the child away from artificial colors and preservatives in foods. My son tried Ritalin for about a year in the early 1970s but positive effects didn't last. He was helped more by Dr. Feingold's diet changes. However, I couldn't accept Feingold's secondary list of foods to avoid. These included all those with natural bright colors like berries, cherries and tomatoes. Feingold said they contained salicylates, as does aspirin. Perhaps too crude a chemical test was used to make that assessment. We now know these colored flavones, polyphenols and lycopenes are important antioxidants. Since they have a phenol ring similar to that of salicylic acid, they might have tested like salicylates because of it.

Ritalin continues to be one of the most prescribed drugs for children

Another early theory was to increase natural light in the classroom to decrease hyperactivity. A newer study is needed for students with hyperactivity and attention deficit disorder to see if they respond to a change in diet or better light. It might be easier to give a child Ritalin, but what is the long-term effect? Dr. Mary Ann Block is one of several experts and parents who say that Ritalin has been over-prescribed. She thinks the possibility of food allergies should be addressed first before putting an active child on a powerful chemical. One study indicates that Ritalin acts on the same part of the brain as cocaine acts. Will the child who takes Ritalin for many years permanently alter his brain chemistry and be more likely to get addicted to cocaine?

Apparently normal children might be harmed in subtle ways by manufactured foods. Even if the chemical additives and the high sugar content don't cause allergies or hyperactivity, the child who eats junk food might become the adult with food cravings, possibly altered brain chemistry and a tendency for obesity. It's hard to combat advertising for sweet, colored cereals and artificially colored soft drinks. It's up to you as parents to see that your children consume wholesome natural food and drink.

The fact that most authors list wheat as one of the principle allergens and sugar as one of the substances that can alter brain chemistry explains why most manufactured food should be shunned as junk. Even using different theories, the Diamonds and Gittleman also advise against sugary or starchy manufactured foods. You can stop buying sweet, colored soft drinks and other manufactured junk food. Your children will be healthier and slimmer. You will lose weight and not have to take prescription drugs to repair your brain chemistry. Your mental attitude can improve without stimulants. You won't continually crave carbohydrates if you stay away from foods that might be causing allergies or addictions.

For many years, doctors prescribed thyroid hormones and/or stimulants for overweight people

It often didn't work. If people with adequate thyroid hormones take extra, their own thyroid gland makes less. Dr. Schwarzbein, Ross and others say only certain people need thyroid medication. Stimulants like ephedra, given to increase metabolism of fat, made some patients feel tired but wired. Their bodies and brains were like an underfed overworked horse that is whipped when it doesn't go fast enough. Drugs and stimulants might relieve symptoms in the short-term, but if the basic problems remain, you won't get healthy and you'll regain fat. You can't rely on a quick fix. You took a long time to put on fat and you must work diligently to lose it.

If you are tired of staying fat, despite dieting, see if you're sensitive to certain foods

Dr. Elson Haas' book is good for the moderately obese to find out if an allergy or food sensitivity is causing uncomfortable false fat. Dr. Rivas is good in correlating personality traits to brain chemicals for anyone who fails on regular diets, even though he is too pessimistic by requiring life-long medication or supplements. Dr. Schwarzbein shows that a diet moderately high in protein and fat can reverse eating disorders that lead to obesity and other metabolic disease. She says to omit junk foods and artificial stimulants. Dr. Lesser shows the relationship of brain chemistry to faulty diets that result in negative moods or behavioral problems even if weight loss isn't necessary.

Most of the above authors think amino acids can correct deficiencies in the major brain chemicals such as serotonin, nor-epinephrine and dopamine. They can also help people addicted to carbohydrates. A diet high in good quality meat, cottage cheese, eggs, soy and wheat germ might be better than either prescription drugs or expensive supplements as the life-long cure of obesity.

Ross' book *The Diet Cure*, with its detailed 12-week plan to repair brain chemistry and normalize hormones, seems the best book to recommend for the seriously overweight person. You might want to start with the high amounts of amino acids advised by Julia Ross. You might follow Dr. Lesser's advice on using vitamins, specific amino acids and other supplements in addition to a good natural diet after an analysis of brain chemicals and minerals in your blood. Your doctor might prescribe the drugs Dr. Rivas uses. It took many years for you to alter your metabolism and it might take months to get your body so it can make enough of all the chemicals needed by your brain. Then you won't continually crave the foods you shouldn't have.

You have the power to change the level of certain chemicals in your brain

You may have to give up addicting foods and use certain amino acids as well as a higher protein diet. A later chapter shows how brain chemistry improves with exercise. No diet works in the long run without increased activity. You can overcome food addictions and avoid debilitating aging by gaining good health. Just losing fat is not enough.

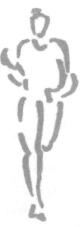

What You Can Do

- First eliminate wheat, milk, sugar, eggs, corn, soy and peanuts to see if bloating and false fat go away. Add each of the foods back for a week and see which causes the false fat to return.

- See if specific foods make your pulse rate increase.

- If you continually crave and eat carbohydrate foods, it's probably an addiction. You might be one of the millions of people who should never eat sugars and most starches.

- Always have a protein food with meals and snacks to get a variety of amino acids. Nuts, seeds and cheese are good snacks.

- Eat lots of vegetables, lesser amounts of fruit and plenty of both animal and plant proteins. Use truly whole-grain products, but only those which don't cause allergy or intolerance.

- Avoid all manufactured foods and beverages. Besides sugar and wheat, unnatural substances in these products can cause metabolic problems as well as obesity and possible allergies.

- If you occasionally fail and eat something you know isn't good for you, forgive yourself and then get back on the right track.

- Besides cutting out stimulants, sugar and other sensitizing foods, you need to change your lifestyle. Obesity is a symptom, not a cause of disease. There aren't any instant easy methods. Prepare for the long haul and keep trying to improve your health.

- Aim for a Golden Mean between the one extreme of your present habits, which aren't working, and the other extreme of becoming dependent on the life-long use of prescription drugs.

Extreme Diets & Some Other Programs

There's a clever folk song about a cat that someone tried to get rid of. No matter what extreme measures the owner took, the cat came back. We need a similar ditty about how a person tried all sorts of pills, diets and injections to lose weight but the fat came back.

Quick fix diets don't last or have these side-effects.

Harvey had been taking prescription drugs for weight loss. When the news came out that heart problems were caused by fen-phen (fenfluramine and phentermine), his doctor didn't renew his prescription. Harvey then tried human growth hormone injections to lose his pot belly. It worked as long as he was getting that expensive product. When he stopped the injections and continued with his usual diet and activities, the fat came back.

Recent diet books and older ones recommend different ratios of protein, carbohydrate and fat

Some authors are extreme in advising what to avoid for their weight loss program. How can you decide what to limit if not total calories? You might have tried all the various systems already and always gained back the fat you lost. I'll point out pitfalls in the extreme diets and mention some moderate diets that have minor drawbacks. You'll be ready for the next chapter Diets for Health.

I remember reading a fanciful satire by a confused fellow medical student. He wrote that he didn't want to eat proteins because they might give him gout. He didn't want to eat carbohydrates because they might give him diabetes. He didn't want to eat fats because they might make him too fat. He decided the only way to survive would be to inject chlorophyll in his veins and lie in the sun to make all his nutrients just like a plant does. They use the raw materials carbon dioxide, water and minerals to make all the carbohydrates, proteins and fats they need.

Of course, photosynthesis is impossible in a human, but what is the answer for an ideal healthy diet? In the last 60 or 70 years, diseases such as diabetes, heart disease, stroke and cancer have been increasing. Even in the past 30 years, though many people have quit smoking and cut down on eating fat, these diseases haven't gone away. In fact, diabetes and obesity have increased dramatically.

Dr. Irwin Stillman's book , Quick Weight Loss Diet, was known as the meat and water diet

A write-up in Parade magazine in the 1960s showed one of his patients telling how easy it was to lose weight with his method. The accompanying photographs disturbed me. The "before" picture was of a healthy-looking man with a round face and some extra fat. In the "after" picture he looked gaunt with dry, furrowed skin. Nevertheless, along with my friends I tried the diet. Most of us did lose weight. The one who didn't lose got very little exercise. I remember seeing her in her nightgown cleaning the oven, since she restricted herself to climbing stairs only once or twice a day. Perhaps members of the cat family don't lose weight on an all-meat diet because they lie around 20 to 23 hours a day. All of us who tried the diet had some coarsening of our features like the man in the Parade article.

On Dr. Stillman's diet, I lost several pounds in two weeks; it came off much more slowly after that. It was the first time since the birth of my second child I weighed less than 135 pounds. Then one knee began to hurt when I did deep knee bends, but nothing unusual was seen on the x-ray. However, the creatinine and uric acid levels in my blood were higher than normal. The doctor said that if my uric acid got any higher, I could get gout and might need medication. Knowing that too much meat had caused the abnormalities in my blood tests, I cut way back. I started a more balanced diet containing fruit, vegetables, whole-grain bread and nuts. These foods plus carrot and celery juice helped me get back to normal. I could again do knee bends without pain.

Besides being unbalanced, the meat and water diet had lots of unavoidable animal fat. About that time, we heard that the fat of animals might contain insecticides, antibiotics and hormones. When we ate meat, these substances were passed on to us and stored in our body fat. Before DDT was banned, a poster showed a pregnant woman and stated that her breast milk would be unhealthy for her baby because of the DDT it probably contained. After we heard reports of the deaths of amateur athletes who were on the very unbalanced Stillman diet, nobody I knew stayed on it. Later, other scientists said the early weight loss on this diet was water along with muscle proteins.

Another extreme diet of about 30 years ago suggested oils to curb your appetite

It advised sipping from a small wineglass of vegetable oil at a party instead of drinking a cocktail. The oil would take away your desire to eat any hors d'oeuvres or the main meal. One woman who tried it said it took away her appetite by making her nauseous. Obviously that diet didn't catch on.

Nathan Pritikin's no-fat diet was at the other extreme

He thought that even natural plant foods such as nuts, olives and avocados were unhealthy because they contained fat. He said that to get healthy and avoid heart attacks, you should not eat fat of any kind. Having been stung once by an unbalanced diet, I was leery of this extreme no-fat diet. Pritikin's diet and the suggested lifestyle changes did help some men. After the first heart attack, they knew their lives were at stake. They finally quit smoking, did vigorous exercise and ate lots of vegetables as well as staying away from fat. The other items in the total program probably did more good than cutting out fat. However, most people thought that eating no fat was most important.

About that time the vegetarian "Diet for a Small Planet" made a lot of sense

The author, Frances M. Lappe, paired foods like corn and beans which complemented each other to provide a complete mixture of all the essential amino acids in each meal. This diet appealed to many young people who became vegetarians. As the world gets smaller with rapidly increasing populations, it makes sense to eat low on the food chain. It takes a lot of land and water to raise animals for food. My father, who was in the U.S. Forest Service in Colorado, said it took 20 or more acres of range-land to raise one steer. With the present factory farms, less land but more water is used. In soils where grain and soybeans can be grown, it is less wasteful for humans to eat these products directly instead of feeding it to animals.

However, some of the vegetarian recipes from the book I made for the family caused gas and others were too complicated. When my older son left home, he became a vegetarian, subsisting mainly on beans and rice. When I spent a month with him, I added eggs and cheese as well as vegetables and fruit. We both felt energetic and did a lot of hiking, causing me to lose weight.

Fiber in food is necessary for permanent weight loss and optimum health

In 1975, *Dr. Sanford Siegal's Natural Fiber Permanent Weight Loss Diet* noted that whenever primitive people adopted a typical western diet, they started getting the diseases of civilization including obesity, diabetes and heart disease. He had charts showing the ratio of carbohydrate to the fiber content in foods (C/F value). He said to avoid foods with a very high value such as cakes and puddings, and to add bran to foods with a moderately high C/F value.

All cereals aren't equal. Cooked oatmeal has a C/F of 44 while cream of wheat has a C/F of 247. Most cereal flakes have values near 100 and sugar-coated cereals are off the chart, as are most cookies, cakes and fruit juices. He said you could improve a basic American diet by adding bran to various foods. For example, use it instead of bread crumbs in meat loaf and add it to baked goods. Too much bran caused gas in some people, even when they started gradually as Siegal recommends. Adding bran doesn't make a poor diet nutritious anyway.

Most experts now say we all must eat more fiber. One author is extreme, saying that women should consume 20 to 35 grams of fiber and men 30 to 50 grams per day. (An ounce is 28 grams.) An apple with skin or a potato with skin has 4 grams of fiber, as does a cup of cooked brown rice or an ounce of bran cereal. Other authors say six to seven servings of these or similar foods should be sufficient for the lesser amounts of 25 to 30 grams they recommend. Most agree that it's best to get it as the naturally occurring fiber in vegetables, fruits and unrefined grain products. Adding bran to a deficient diet or stirring up a glass of some substance that is supposed to keep you regular isn't as good. You need the other nutrients and micro-nutrients of natural foods.

Fiber isn't a single substance. Insoluble fiber or cellulose helps the movement of materials through the intestine. Soluble fiber includes lignin, the pectin in apples and other fruits and the component of oat bran that absorbs cholesterol in the intestine and carries it out of the body. You can find bins of granola in groceries as well as in health food stores. Basic granola is oatmeal baked with oil and honey or brown sugar. It is better than puffy, crunchy or candy-like prepared cereals because of the natural oat fiber. High-fiber diets were a start in the right direction but not the whole answer for healthy eating.

By the 1980s, many people had adopted a low-fat, high-carbohydrate diet

It was often low in protein. It worked for many athletes. Gone were the training tables that had lots of meat and milk. It didn't make sense for athletes to tax their livers and kidneys to convert protein foods into energy for competition. Before strenuous exercise, it was better to eat foods that were either high in glucose or readily converted to it, such as bread and pasta. But advocates of a high-carbohydrate, low-protein diet ignored the need for dietary protein to repair muscles after the exercise was finished. Even less active adults need some protein; growing children need a lot of it. Everyone needs natural fatty acids for new cell walls. Even saturated fat will replenish body fat burned during strenuous sustained exercise. Fat and cholesterol are necessary for the immune system and to make hormones.

Ordinary people found that a diet good for athletes caused them to gain fat instead of losing it. Many American women of the time ate 43 percent of their calories as fat, 46 percent as carbohydrate and 11 percent as protein. They reduced fats and increased carbohydrates as recommended by the media as well as many doctors. It wasn't a good weight loss diet. One-quarter of Americans were overweight in 1975, but by 2001 this figure had increased to half and continues to grow.

Robert Pritikin, son of the founder of the Pritikin Longevity Center, wrote a book aimed at the average person

His book, *Pritikin Weight Loss Breakthrough,* does advocate a little fat but emphasizes natural fiber. Even with complex carbohydrates that are absorbed slowly, it is necessary to eat six times a day to avoid feeling hungry. The more you exercise, the more you crave carbohydrates. As your glycogen reserves get depleted, you must continue to eat more carbohydrate. He says to limit consumption of animal foods to 3½ ounces per day - for example: two small servings of skim milk cheese, or about 4 percent of a 1,600 calorie diet. Beans can provide additional protein but very high amounts of carbohydrates predominate. It is still a very unbalanced diet. Without enough fat and protein, it's no wonder people always feel hungry on this diet.

In contrast, Dr. Robert Atkins said to eat more protein and little or no carbohydrate

Modifying Dr. Stillman's diet, Atkins' plan evolved over time.

Dr. Atkin's New Diet Revolution was a best seller concerning weight loss. The later *Dr. Atkin's Age-Defying Diet* uses similar principles and correlates the factors that make a person obese with those related to diabetes, heart disease and cancer. Atkins advises eating a very high-protein diet with no carbohydrates at the beginning of his weight loss program. You gradually add more carbohydrate. After reaching your desired weight, you can eat 30 percent protein, 30 percent fat and 40 percent carbohydrate. It is often hard to stay on his early weight loss diet. Overweight people I've talked with lost some weight without feeling hungry but quit long before they got to the balanced maintenance phase. They missed carbohydrate foods, especially bread. Artificial bread made with egg whites is more like a meringue and can't take the place of bread.

Dr. Atkin's Diet and diabetes

Two unrelated acquaintances, in their thirties, have been on the Atkins diet for several months. Both had developed type II diabetes after gaining a lot of weight. Karen was afraid of needles and asked her doctor if she could try Dr. Atkins high-protein diet instead of starting insulin. He said it would probably be all right for a month or two, then to go on a more balanced diet. Several months later, Karen was still plump but she didn't need insulin. She looked marvelous and can now wear skirts with a waistline instead of fancy muumuus. She will slowly lose more weight.

Kirk said he lost 40 pounds in a few months after he read Dr. Atkins' book. He will keep using the most restrictive phase of the diet. His blood sugar is down and he says he's glad he won't have to face the deadly effects of diabetes. He still has a large abdomen but thinks he can get rid of it within a year by continuing Atkins' weight-loss diet.

This seems like too long a time to be without the two kinds of fiber and the vitamins, minerals and antioxidants in fruits, vegetables and whole-grain products. Karen is taking a better approach. People like Kirk use Dr. Atkins book as a bible, not questioning whether the extreme early diet might have unforeseen effects over a long-term before reaching the healthier maintenance phase.

Several authors say a high-protein, low-carbohydrate diet is unhealthy

Robert Haas, in his book *Eat to Win*, has no use for the "protein pushers." He calls his a "Mediter-Asian" diet, using a variety of vegetarian foods from other cultures. However, in order to stay healthy, he says you need many juices and special drinks with a variety of supplements in addition to food. He says to lose weight, get your carbohydrates from fruits and vegetables but eat only two servings of a grain product a day. This may be a thin slice of bread or a small serving of oatmeal or brown rice. Most of his proteins come from soybean products.

He concedes that low fat diets don't work in the long run. His maintenance diet has 15 percent fat along with 25 percent protein and 60 percent carbohydrate. This is more moderate than Pritikin's approach but requires lots of daily exercise and more dedication than the typical American has. Most of us are neither competitive athletes nor the Hollywood celebrities who have followed the Haas diet. It seems that authors who most strongly advise a high carbohydrate diet say you should run or do similar aerobic exercise at least an hour a day, six days a week. Jane Fonda says she bicycles or does other exercise two hours a day.

In *Dr. Bob Arnot's Revolutionary Weight Control Program*, Arnot touts a diet heavy in fiber especially beans. It has no saturated fat and a minimum amount of olive oil or canola oil. He says to concentrate on hard foods to get a hard, lean body since foods that are hard to chew require longer digestion. Soybeans are his favorite snack. Arnot thinks that whole-wheat pasta cooked *al dente* will be absorbed slower than ordinary white pasta. He says to avoid anything made with refined white flour, to which most health-conscious people would agree. In contrast to Haas, Arnot says, "Fruit juice is to fruit as white flour is to whole-grain." [Besides fiber, whole fruit has bioflavonoids and other micronutrients.]

Arnot believes protein intake should vary with the level of activity. However, even with five levels he classifies together as level one, both a sedentary person and one who does less than forty minutes of aerobic exercise a day. A 120-pound woman would get 44 grams of protein each day, and a 180-pound man 65 grams. These calculate out as 10 to 12 percent protein. This seems low even for a sedentary person, and certainly low for someone exercising moderately. Of course, it's wasteful to use protein as an energy source but we all need it to make enzymes, repair cells and keep a healthy immune system.

Arnot's diet would be too high in carbohydrate and too low in protein and fat for most people. Like Pritikin, he recommends three snacks as well as three meals a day along with one or more exercise sessions each day. Does the average person have that much time to follow a rigid schedule built around eating and exercise periods? Can many people adhere to it throughout life?

A rigid ascetic approach doesn't work in the long run

Andrew Weil, M.D., author of *Eating Well for Optimum Health*, thinks that meals should be enjoyable and preferably social times. He advocates 50 to 100 grams protein on a 2,000-calorie-a-day diet. This works out to about 10 to 20 percent protein. Weil says that up to 30 percent of calories can come from three types of fat in the ratio of 1: 2: 1 of saturated fat: mono-unsaturated fat: poly-unsaturated fat. Eat cheese, butter and eggs for saturated fat, olive oil for the mono-unsaturated and the oil in fatty fish for the poly-unsaturated fat. His regimen sounds more like a true Mediter-Asian diet with cheese and fish as well as fruits and vegetables. With 30 percent fat, 15 to 20 percent protein and 50 to 55 percent carbohydrate it is a moderate diet that most people could follow.

Barry Sears says to balance carbohydrate with adequate protein and fat

In his book, *The Zone*, Sears says that a so-called "healthy diet" of 70 percent carbohydrate, 15 percent protein and 15 percent fat is to blame for most obesity. Extreme vegetarian diets with 80 percent carbohydrate and 10 percent each of fat and protein are even worse. Sears calls his the "zone diet." It has 30 percent fat, 30 percent protein and 40 percent carbohydrate. His idea is to make a balanced ratio of about 3 grams of protein for every 4 grams of carbohydrates. This keeps the body in a healthy zone between a high blood sugar that stimulates too much insulin and an excess of protein that leads to the incomplete burning of fat. You would adjust protein depending on activity level. In my chapter on insulin and other hormones you learned that glucagon, a second pancreatic hormone, is stimulated by protein. It opposes and normalizes the action of insulin. Sears' balanced ratio is good but some of his recommendations are too low in total calories.

The Protein Power diet

Drs. Michael and Mary Dan Eades in *Protein Power* advocate more protein. This is based on your ideal body weight, not your present weight. A 120-pound woman should have 70 grams protein per day and a 180-pound man needs 100 grams. Protein foods contain from 3 to 7 grams of actual protein per ounce (28 grams). Meat has 7 grams per ounce, eggs 6 grams per ounce, hard cheese 6-7 grams per ounce, soft cheeses 3-4 grams per ounce and tofu 5 grams per ounce. Each person should also have 25 grams of fiber and 30 to 55 grams of carbohydrate. [This is very low even for a beginning reducing diet.] Dietary fat should be high quality, from seeds, nuts, olive oil or butter and never from margarine or other trans fats. [I explained trans fats in the section on body chemistry.]

The Eades' later book, *The Protein Power Life Plan*, tells more about increasing protein and limiting carbohydrate to combat metabolic diseases like diabetes as well as obesity. An important chapter in their book emphasizes getting enough magnesium. Others tell the importance of good quality fats and cholesterol. It is well researched and more comprehensive than Atkins' books. It gives three levels of diet suggestions, depending on how closely you want to simulate the healthy diet of Paleolithic man. All have adequate protein and limited carbohydrates.

Several authors list carbohydrates according to a glycemic index

This indicates how quickly the starch becomes glucose with a value of 100. Whole wheat bread has a value of 70 and oatmeal 49. Many fruits and root vegetables are between 40 and 70. The lower the value, the slower it gets into your blood stream as glucose to raise your insulin and make you hungry again.

The Doctors Eades classify carbohydrate foods more stringently, only subtracting fiber carbohydrates from total carbohydrates in a food since our bodies can't digest them. They talk about effective carbohydrate content (ECC). Sugars and all starches are lumped into one category, since they all end up as glucose, though at different rates of digestion. Forget whether a food tastes sweet or not. Half a cup of cooked carrots has 4.3 grams of effective carbohydrate even though they taste sweet. Beans have 20 to 22 grams, about like a sweet potato at 24 grams. Remember, these ECC values are sugars plus starches.

Are all these grams and percentages confusing?

You really don't need to use a bunch of charts to calculate the grams of carbohydrate, protein and fat in your food. You probably should not read labels. Packaged and canned foods list calories and percentages of these nutrients in their products. They can mislead people to eat more carbohydrates since they have 4 calories per gram as compared to 9 in fat. How many people have the time or incentive to read labels and make all those calculations? You don't need to figure calories or grams of carbohydrate, protein or fat if you get all three in a wide variety of natural foods, including many servings of vegetables.

The diets with the most failures have been too low in total calories. You lose weight quickly by losing muscle. Then your metabolism slows down and it gets hard to lose fat and easy to put it back on. But pick up any magazine and you see another low-calorie diet often low in fiber, with juices, not whole foods. They are also very low in fat, another reason you feel hungry all the time and eventually go on a binge of high-calorie foods.

Most processed foods are high in carbohydrates

Much of the obesity of the past 30 years has been from the huge increase in eating processed foods. The old USDA food pyramid didn't help. It advocates 10 or more servings of grain products, including pasta, daily. Many prepackaged foods advertised as low in fat have high levels of carbohydrates, along with many non-nutritive chemicals. White rice, pasta and most breads have starch carbohydrates that are easily changed into glucose. The body treats them as simple sugars.

The 2005 USDA food pyramid now says that healthy complex carbohydrates are whole-grain products. They take longer to digest and contain the vitamins, minerals and fiber of the original grain. Oatmeal is the best known. Other complex carbohydrates exist in potatoes, yams, beans and root vegetables. Whole-grain loaves of bread are often firm. Many don't contain additives like most commercial bread, so are best bought unsliced to prevent mold. It's easy to make very thin slices as you need them.

Should we change with each theory about what is healthy or harmful?

Some diet ideas are based on a faulty understanding of physiology. Others apply to athletes or people with specific problems. The media and advertisers generalize and apply them to everyone. We are individuals with different body types and activity levels. It's interesting that authors who strongly advise a high-carbohydrate diet are the ones who say you should run or do similar aerobic exercise at least an hour a day, six days a week. The high carbohydrate diet of a runner is not appropriate for someone sitting at a desk all day. If you subtract the calories used in running and count those when a runner is sedentary, percentages of fat, protein and carbohydrate will be closer to that of authors who recommend less carbohydrate. Subtract the 700 calories expended in the day's running from a 2,000 calorie diet that is 70 percent carbohydrate, 15 percent protein and 15 percent fat. Recalculate on the basis of 1,300 calories and get 53 percent carbohydrate, 23 percent protein and 23 percent fat. This is closer to the 40 percent: 30 percent: 30 percent of Barry Sears and others who think women especially should eat more protein.

The Atkins diet goes too far in the other direction. You get too much protein and little or no carbohydrate for many months. A high-meat diet can cause other problems. Meat is plentiful in the U.S. so more people have started the Atkins diet. Meat prices have gone down in the past 40 years, so more people have it often. Chicken or beef used to be special and served for Sunday dinner. Chicken is no longer a luxury. It was the first meat raised in enough quantities to be cheap for the consumer. Chickens make more efficient use of the grain they're fed than do larger animals. Also, their wastes can be used as fertilizer.

However, in the past decade or two, factory farms growing pork and beef have sprung up in many parts of the country. The average working man will eat cheaper steaks and hamburgers and take his chances with his health. He doesn't worry about how his meat was raised so long as he can eat it every day. Factory farms produce a prodigious amount of waste. It is so concentrated that if it were spread on the ground it would burn any crops one tried to grow. It can only be kept in lagoons for bacteria to slowly change some of it into less noxious compounds. Some complex chemicals such as hormones or antibiotics might not break down. The cheap availability of meat has other costs. Have you ever smelled a factory animal farm? It isn't pleasant.

Just as with Dr. Stillman's meat and water diet of 40 years ago, the absence of carbohydrates does cause weight loss. At first, this is mainly from water and the breakdown of proteins to make the blood glucose necessary for brain metabolism. Since muscle weighs more than fat, the person weighs less even when little body fat is metabolized. After a few days body fat is used, but not burned completely, often causing a person's breath to smell like acetone.

Eating large amounts of supermarket meat can be harmful to your health

Dr. Michael Pollan spoke on public radio about his article

on factory beef farms in the October 12, 2003 issue of the *New York Times*, titled "The (Agricultural Contradictions of Obesity." Ranchers in the early 1900s took four to six years to grow a steer big enough to sell. Their sons could bring a grass-fed steer to market in two to three years by taking it to a feed lot to spend the last month eating corn. This short-term corn-fed beef used to be considered prime, with a marbling of fat between muscle fibers. Now, in the factory farms a marketable 250-pound steer takes 14 to 16 months to mature; it is fed corn the entire time after weaning.

Pollan talked of animal cities where 100,000 cattle are crowded together to eat tons of corn and some soybeans. For quicker weight gain, they get a pellet of estrogen implanted under their skin. They also need antibiotics. In fact, for the past 50 years, half of all antibiotics went to livestock to kill the bacteria in their intestines so more of their feed was used to put on weight. Confining the animals makes it more necessary to use insecticides and additional antibiotics to control disease.

Corn is concentrated feed, easy to transport and subsidized by the government. At $2.50 a bushel, it's cheaper than hay. In order to raise that much corn, farmers use large amounts of fertilizer, mainly ammonium nitrate made from petroleum — 1.2 gallons of oil to produce one bushel of corn, according to Pollan. This raises the yield per acre so much that an organic farmer can't compete. Cheap subsidized corn helps big agribusiness but doesn't make Americans healthier.

Additionally, a corn diet goes against the natural metabolism of the steers. Cattle are ruminants. They partially digest grass then bring it up as a cud to chew. This material then goes to another section of stomach, the rumen, where special bacteria digest the cellulose in the grass and produce proteins. In order to get to market faster, cattle in feed lots never get hay, only the cheap, subsidized corn. Since their metabolism developed over millennia to digest grass, they get an unnatural fermentation in a bloated rumen. Acidified products can cause lesions in the rumen and other harmful bacteria are carried to the liver.

According to Pollan, 13 percent of feed-lot cattle have liver abscesses despite the use of extra antibiotics. Just as over-use of antibiotics in humans has caused resistant strains of bacteria to develop, the same is true with livestock. *E. coli* 0157, a lethal strain in hamburger, only appears in feed-lot cattle. It's no wonder Europeans don't want our meat.

Much of the meat at markets has been grown in factory farms

The fat formed between muscle fibers is eaten by the consumer. Other fat is ground into hamburger. Your body fat has collected too many fat-soluble toxic chemicals already. The combination of releasing these as you lose body fat along with adding more toxins from your diet into your system is not healthy. Don't make the mistake of going from 80 percent of your calories as carbohydrates to the other extreme of zero or very low carbohydrates and too much protein.

Low-carb. processed foods might be as bad for you as low-fat processed foods. These manufactured foods might still contain an array of unnatural ingredients including trans fats and high-fructose corn syrup. The dangers from these were discussed in earlier chapters. Some chemical sweeteners might be safe over a short period unless you're allergic to them. Aspartame, though widely used, can cause adverse reactions in some people. The Doctors Eades say only the herbal product Stevia is safe for long-term use.

Don't stay on the very restricted Atkins weight-loss diet more than a month or two. Too much meat can be unhealthy. It can cause gout and other metabolic problems. The high phosphorus in meat can draw calcium from your bones and cause osteoporosis. Don't think that just taking calcium pills will prevent this. As explained in other chapters, calcium pills can go through your digestive system unabsorbed. You need a well-balanced diet with adequate protein, not all of it from meat. In fact, a recent advertisement of the Atkins Food Pyramid shows only the later maintenance phase. This includes foods containing carbohydrate. It pictures eggs, fish, shell fish, tofu and chicken at the base of the pyramid. It doesn't show red meat but mentions beef and pork in the text. These are the products that consumers are now buying in larger amounts. Many people are eating a big steak with salad, like what we thought was the ideal meal in the 1960s.

One friend recently devised his own extreme diet. He ate nothing all day and for dinner had a big salad containing a diced chicken breast and some olive oil. He did lose pounds but not evenly. Six months later, his abdomen was still prominent.

Another friend described a woman who lost 100 pounds on the Atkins diet. However, she ended up with lots of loose flesh. Even though her fat cells are empty, they're still there. Now she faces extensive surgery in order to remove the flab. Without a good balanced diet, it will take longer for surgical incisions to heal and she might get unsightly scars. Even if she's not fat, she is still not healthy. People who lose fat by liposuction aren't healthy either, unless they exercise and change their dietary habits. Thinness does not automatically equal health.

A point of agreement in all the diets is to avoid processed foods. We are hooked on junk food and advertisers make sure we remain junkies. Packaged low-carb snacks are still junk food.

In summary, avoid extreme diets. They are all missing one or more ingredients essential to health. Liquid diets don't have fiber. The Pritikin diet is missing fat and is low in protein. The Haas and Arnot diets are too high in carbohydrates. The Atkins diet is too high in protein and lacks essential fruits and vegetables for many months.

Eat natural foods and get moderate amounts of protein, fat and carbohydrates Natural foods with little processing give you fiber and some carbohydrate but not too much. Just as your heart and other muscles prefer to burn fats, your brain needs glucose, best obtained from the metabolism of carbohydrate foods. Also, during vigorous exercise an old adage might be true: Fat burns best in the flame of carbohydrates.

What You Can Do

- Forget the promises of quick weight loss that comes with any extreme diet.

- You can aim for the Golden Mean by going to the following chapter on Diets for Better Health, and using one of the alternative diet pyramids or other programs described there.

- All of these are superior to the USDA food pyramid. These will help you to get healthier and maintain your best body weight.

- Other chapters will discuss vitamins, minerals and other supplements to a good diet.

- Review the chapter on allergies and food intolerance where the authors tell how you can alter chemicals in your brain to get rid of cravings that control you and make you fat.

- Later chapters emphasize exercise that you can continue the rest of your life.

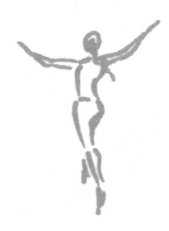

Diets for
Better Health

If you're in the normal range according to the
Body Mass Index, you want to delay aging.
You can keep or regain some of the energy and
body proportions of youth.

If you're overweight or obese, you want to lose fat. You first need to commit to a lifetime of health, no matter how long it takes to see results. Quick weight loss by one of the extreme diets described earlier won't do it.

You are ready to consider a healthy diet you can follow the rest of your life

Excess body fat is a symptom, not a cause of disease. Liposuction or an extreme diet might remove fat or produce a lower weight, but it doesn't make you healthy. You need a diet of natural foods that contain fat as well as carbohydrates and proteins. After showing the problems of the average American diet, I will present alternatives as guidelines. You can change your diet and your lifestyle to become fit and trim.

Americans are eating less fat but getting fatter partly because of eating more total calories

According to Marion Nestle in the book *Food Politics: How the Food Industry Influences Nutrition and Health,* 320,000 different food products are made every year. If all were sold, that would be 3,800 calories for every person every day, including children and the elderly. Since only some professional athletes or lumberjacks need that much, the companies are spending billions of dollars to get consumers to eat more of their products. They use colorful advertisements on television or offer schools and other organizations big money to stock only their brand of soft drinks in the vending machines and/or serve them in the cafeteria. Many children are drinking more soft drinks than milk. One mother I know says kids are so used to soft drinks that at parties most mothers serve soft drinks with the birthday cake instead of milk.

Sweet liquids go down easily just like water

However, a 64-ounce soft drink can contain 800 calories. This could represent one-third to one-half of the total daily calories needed by a sedentary person. When I accompanied three hiking friends into a fast food outlet, I noticed the exhibit of large 32- to 48-ounce cups with the names of various soft drinks along with a sign that read: "Get a free refill when you buy any of these." Nestle says the sugar lobby got the USDA food pyramid to change "limit" to "moderate" your sugar intake. Two quarts of sugary pop is excessive for anybody.

The USDA food pyramid had replaced the basic four food groups of good nutrition

At the base of the pyramid are bread, cereals, pasta and potatoes. Next come fruits and vegetables with five to seven servings a day. Then moderate dairy and meat followed by oils and sweets at the top of the pyramid. The new pyramid, out in 2005 is somewhat better. It advises using whole-grains, but still suggests 6-11 servings daily. Fats, oils and sweets should be used sparingly. It says to use low-fat milk, cheese or yogurt and to prepare meat to get rid of fat. It says choose fewer foods high in sugars (not much of a warning, compared to fat).

Moreover, many Americans think that pasta and noodles are no different from prepackaged foods they see at the supermarket, such as bright orange macaroni and cheese, various cereals, cookies, crackers and other snacks. Since they're based on grain, they must be good for you. Wrong. Only whole-grain products contain fiber, so are true complex carbohydrates. Products made from refined flour, such as pasta, bread and most cereals, are easily turned into glucose and act like sugar to raise the insulin level in your blood.

The starches in most manufactured foods aren't better than sugars. Worst are foods with added high-fructose corn syrup. As shown in an earlier chapter, the liver changes fructose into fat and LDL cholesterol.

Studies of the Western diet ignore the sugars in soft drinks and starches in packaged foods

Most just point out the addition of more meat in a westernized diet. Human beings have been eating fat meat and eggs for millennia. Sugar consumption 300 years ago was only a few pounds a year. In the twentieth century, it rose steadily in the U.S. to 100 pounds a year in 1970. It is now almost 150 pounds per person per year.

Ethnic diets can vary from region to region in the same country. When I visited south India in 1996, I noticed that throughout, the main starches were either rice or some type of wheat-based flat bread. Most often lentils or chick-peas furnished the needed protein. In some areas, people ate eggs or chicken. The people looked healthiest in the villages near the sea where fish markets were replete with many types of fish. Obesity was rare in the villages and cities I visited in the state of Karnataka and most of Maharashtra, including Bombay. I did see more fat people in the city of Ahmedabad in the state of Gujerat. You can't buy beer there so people drink more soft drinks. People in all walks of life in Gujerat consume much more sugar than in other states. In most of India, sugar might be used only to sweeten the morning tea—less than 15 pounds per person per year.

American sugar-lovers resist thinking that using sugar might have consequences

One friend countered my preceding observation with one of his own. He had visited Cuba after the fall of the USSR in the early 1990s. He said when the Russians were no longer providing oils, the Cubans ate more sugar and were thin as rails. Even babies who got cane juice instead of milk weren't fat. To me this indicates a lack of total calories, not that sugars are benign and can't be changed into fat.

When I was a child, desserts were common at both lunch and dinner. My father had grown up on a farm; sweets helped provide energy for hard work in the fields. Many Americans have similar forebears and expect desserts once or twice daily. Their ancestors in the old countries might have looked forward to such foods only at holidays.

You needn't give up all sweet foods. Have dessert once a week and really appreciate it. You can gradually lose a sweet tooth. A dessert with dates or raisins can replace a cream pie. Days or weeks later, eat only fresh fruit at the end of a meal. A dessert with an artificial sweetener won't break your sugar habit. It might even make it worse as your taste buds expect more sweetness.

People often think a substance is either good or bad. They need a sense of balance. Eating healthy foods should be a habit, broken only on special occasions. One book from years ago said to keep from gaining weight, avoid the habits of bread and butter, deep-fried foods and daily desserts. It didn't say never to have them. Just don't get in the habit of regularly eating these foods. For today's teens and adults I would add: Never form a soft-drink-habit.

My advice for all ages is: Beware of "easy calories"

Easiest to consume are sweet liquids, especially soft drinks. *Easy calories* are not necessarily empty calories. Fruit juices contain vitamins and minerals as well as sugars, but they are easy to swallow. There is nothing satisfying about these liquids, to remind your body to stop. Milk is the only liquid that turns to a semi-solid when it hits the acid in your stomach. Calories in solid foods that contain fiber, complex carbohydrates, protein or fat are limiting because they make you feel full. Fats have the added advantage of slowing down the emptying time of your stomach.

Most packaged snacks of sugars and starches, often low in fat, give you *easy calories*. Their sugars and starches quickly get into the blood stream. Alcoholic liquids are similar. Again, you don't realize how much you're drinking because those *easy calories* go down and are absorbed so quickly. In addition alcohol yields about seven calories per gram.

Labels on packaged foods imply it doesn't matter what you eat if you limit the calories

They say that fat gives you nine calories per gram and carbohydrate only four calories. They make you think you're okay if you eat foods low in fat. They don't mention the added sugars in their products, more than the former equivalent of fat. Many items are low in fiber so you don't feel you've eaten much even if you have a whole package of snacks.

Stay away from manufactured foods and drinks. These inferior products often contain trans fats and high-fructose corn syrup. These raise your cholesterol and triglycerides and contribute to diabetes and heart disease. It might take months or years for the damage to show, but don't wait.

Concerning meat, the word "moderate" can be as meaningless as the word "serving"

When I was growing up, my mother prepared a pound of round steak. My father got less than five ounces and my mother and we three children got less than three ounces each. It seemed enough. Later in the 1960s, a ten-ounce steak was moderate and a 4-ounce one was tiny. Many restaurant servings are getting larger. Some brag about 24-ounce steaks. For good health, you can enjoy a four to six-ounce piece of meat or fish, something no bigger than your palm.

You need not give up red meat altogether, but aim for quality, not quantity. As mentioned in the chapter on extreme diets, animals grown in factory farms are not healthy. Although you can lose weight without feeling hungry on a high-meat diet, you can't have it the rest of your life without later health problems. Even so-called "organic beef" might mean that the steers got organic corn in the feed-lots. Argentina still raises grass-fed beef, mainly exported to the U.S. for hamburgers, but often mixed with ground meat from factory farms. Michael Pollan states that grass-fed beef contains omega-3 fatty acids and beta-carotene. Corn-fed beef doesn't have these protective factors.

Organic butter or meat should not cause problems

Diet books that advocate eating red meat give the addresses of outlets for grass-fed, organic meat and even sources of wild game. However, these meats cost more and if game animals are raised in crowded feed lots, they aren't superior. "Mad deer" disease, similar to "mad cow" disease, has been found in some game-farm animals.

Warnings about high-protein, low-carbohydrate diets are worth emphasizing. We already covered the dangers of high-carbohydrate, low-fat diets that have been making Americans obese. Again, people want an easy method to shed pounds that doesn't involve strenuous exercise. The absence of carbohydrates does indeed cause weight loss. The body has to remove amino groups from protein products in order to make the blood glucose needed for brain metabolism and quick energy. This inefficient process can use body proteins as well as that from high-protein meals.

A high-meat diet encourages the enlargement of the stomach

The stomach stretches as it churns the meat while adding acid and digestive enzymes. You might have seen pictures of lions or tigers that have just eaten a large amount of meat. Their abdomens are so distended they relax for hours or days until digestion is complete. With protruding bellies, they couldn't catch other prey.

Jim is like a lot of forty-year-olds. He looks well-muscled but does have a pot belly. Jim says that in a recent check-up, he had no indication of diabetes or heart disease. He had normal blood sugar, normal blood lipids and cholesterol. In fact, all his blood tests were normal except for elevated uric acid. I told him that when I was eating lots of meat, my uric acid was high. Very high amounts of uric acid can be deposited near various joints and cause gout, noticed for centuries in wealthy men who ate lots of meat. Increasing vegetables and cutting the size of steaks from

14 or 15 ounces to four or six ounces might help lower uric acid in the blood.

A heavy meat-eater often has a large stomach. If he also eats many desserts, his body will make fat from sugars and deposit this fat around his stomach and other internal organs, giving him a rounded abdomen. (Many people use the word stomach when they mean the abdomen. The stomach is a digestive organ, not an area of the body, properly called the abdomen or belly.) Jim should never start the Atkins diet. He needs to decrease his uric acid, not increase it.

As a vegetarian, Harry is at the opposite extreme. He is thin and sedentary but also has a pot belly. He thinks if he gave up his one beer or one glass of wine a day, he could lose the ten pounds that give him a big waistline. That small amount of alcohol isn't the problem. With both aerobic and resistance exercise, he could get rid of his belly and gain muscle in all parts of his body. He doesn't need a special diet but might increase the amount of total protein, whether from eggs and cheese or plant sources.

The source of the meat is the biggest potential problem with high-protein diets. Much of the meat at the market has been grown in factory farms. This is explained in the chapters on extreme diets and on environmental toxins. With an unnatural high corn diet and over-crowding, these animals are given anti-biotics, insecticides and estrogen to encourage rapid growth and prevent disease. These added substances collect in their fat. The fat formed between muscle fibers is eaten by the consumer. Your body fat has collected too much of these fat-soluble toxic chemicals already. The combination of releasing these as you lose body fat along with adding more toxins from your diet into your system is not good for you.

Some benefits of natural or range-fed beef

Range fed cattle get important omega-3 linolenic acid from green grass into their fat. Thus the best meat is from organic farms or from game animals in natural surroundings. This is more expensive, so it encourages a person to eat smaller portions. Remember, a good daily rule of thumb is to eat a piece of meat smaller or about the size of your palm.

In places where animals are grown naturally, it is safe to eat more than just muscle meat. The French enjoy liver, kidneys, heart and sweetbreads. Consuming the whole animal instead of just eating muscle meat might be a better explanation for the "French Paradox," where the French stay healthy despite eating fat and cholesterol. Nutrients in internal organs might be more important than the popular idea that substances in red wine protect those who consume animal products. In America, liver used to be a valuable source of many nutrients. Now, it contains many chemicals the animal's liver tried to detoxify. Chicken livers, since they're from young birds, are okay to eat once or twice a month. It's too bad that the contaminants in fat and organ meats give them a bad name. This drives many people to eat only skinless chicken and turkey breasts.

Some problems with fish

Fish used to be a good alternative to meat. Now, most freshwater fish should be avoided because of PCBs and mercury in their flesh. Some ocean fish high on the food chain like marlin, shark and tuna also contain many contaminants. I prefer wild salmon from the ocean off Alaska. They are naturally red, while farm-raised salmon are pink, meaning fewer nutrients. Some farm-raised salmon have been treated with a red dye to make them look more appealing. My parents told of an advertising gimmick in the 1930s by a cannery that used inferior salmon: "Our salmon is guaranteed not to turn red in the can." This misleading advertising was soon discredited.

Vegetarians ingest fewer insecticides and require less crop land for their food

Vegetarians stay away from all animal flesh and eat beans, mainly soybeans. True, they get essential amino acids by combining various plant foods, such as beans and corn. Beans, some seeds and nuts can replace meat. Soy protein as in tofu is a complete protein. It can be used in stir-fries or other dishes. Some people, though, are allergic to soy. Others have found it depresses their thyroid gland. Garbanzo beans, also known as chick peas, are excellent. They are used in the Middle East and in Asia. You can make your own *hummus* from chick-pea flour and *tahini* (ground sesame seeds). It makes a lower-calorie spread than peanut butter. One ounce has almost 5 grams protein, less than 3 grams fat and 10 grams carbohydrate. Most peanut butter has 7 grams protein, 14 grams fat and over 6 grams carbohydrate.

Gary Fraser reported on the protective value of nuts in a 1992 study.

The Seventh Day Adventists who ate more nuts had even less cardiovascular disease than others of these low-risk vegetarians. Walnuts are an especially good source of linolenic acid, an omega-3 fatty acid known to prevent cardio-vascular disease. Many seeds and nuts also contain heart-healthy vitamin E. Some contain a good percentage of mono-unsaturated fats like that in olive oil. Many contain linoleic, omega-6 fatty acids. However, both linolenic and linoleic fatty acids are polyunsaturated and can get rancid, so keep your nuts in the refrigerator.

Vegans (eaters of only plant foods) have to take many supplements, especially vitamin B-12, essential in forming red blood cells and nerve tissue. Healthy omnivores make all they need of intracellular substances such as SAMe (S-Adenosylmethionine), alpha lipoic acid, MSM (methyl-sulfo-methane) and other supplements recommended by vegetarian authors. The vegetarians who eat animal products such as eggs or cheese don't need the supplements.

Eggs have more than 6 grams of high-quality protein per egg, along with vitamin A and other nutrients, but only 75 calories each. They are an almost perfect food. But, beware of supermarket eggs produced in factory farms. Best are eggs from free-range chickens. Sometimes they have a thicker shell. Fertile eggs insure that the chickens weren't confined in their individual cubicles but had run around outside in the presence of a rooster.

Vegetarians think they're not getting saturated fat. They get it in their packaged bakery goods or their cream substitute. These often have coconut or palm oils. Worst of all, like most Americans, they get the very bad trans fats in their margarine and bakery goods. The cheapest and worst source is cottonseed oil, because of insecticides used on cotton. Several years ago, we were told to use poly-unsaturated vegetable oils. We now know that they can produce peroxides and free radicals in our bodies. Most poly-unsaturated oils also contain too much omega-6 linoleic acid. Olive oil with its mono-unsaturated fatty acids is the best oil for either vegetarians or omnivores to use on salads and in cooking. Peanut oil and canola oil are all right if kept refrigerated.

Both vegetarians and omnivores need the proper balance of essential fatty acids

Omega-3 can come from flax oil, flax seed, walnuts or fatty cold water fish. Omega-6 can come from most nuts, seeds and their oils. Our ancestors ate a healthy ratio of one part omega-3 (linolenic) to four parts of omega-6 (linoleic) fatty acids. Most modern diets have way too much omega-6 fatty acids, mostly from poly-unsaturated oils in salad dressings, deep-fried foods, margarine and the fats in packaged snack foods and commercial bakery products.

Both vegetarians and meat eaters need to have a healthy ratio, 4:1, of the essential fatty acids, linoleic (omega-6) and linolenic (omega-3) not the 20:1 in most U.S. diets. If the ratio among the three essential fatty acids is correct, don't try to avoid any of them. Cheese and eggs contain a good ratio of 2 percent linoleic and 1 percent linolenic. Egg yolks contain some arachidonic acid. This essential fatty acid has a role in the immune system and in emergency situations. It can be made from the linoleic acid in oils, but this conversion often produces excessive, unhealthy amounts.

Dr. Bob Arnot, in *The Breast Cancer Prevention Diet*, tells patients to stay away from most vegetable oils because they contain omega-6 linoleic acid. He says to avoid most sugars as well. These dietary changes have prevented second cancers in breast cancer survivors.

Vegetarians vary in their degree of health. One vegetarian couple invited me for a spaghetti supper. Their false meatballs, containing cheese, ground-up nuts and mushrooms, were very tasty. They served real butter with the whole-wheat rolls. These vegetarians were of medium weight and their firm smooth skin glowed with health. In contrast, another vegetarian was a very strict vegan. Besides not eating any animal products, he consumed only raw food. He looked like a living skeleton with dry skin and poor muscle tone. Obviously, he was missing a lot of nutrients.

Man is not a gorilla whose body can make all it needs from raw green leaves. Humans cannot be healthy eating nothing but salads.

You must consider the source of any food

Fruit from Chile or Mexico might look beautiful, but if it were grown using DDT or other insecticides banned here, it's not worth buying. Produce at farmer's markets usually has fewer toxic residues than fruits and vegetables in major supermarkets. I don't buy chicken, pork or beef since it is probably from factory farms. Liver, kidneys, heart and sweetbreads (thymus gland) used to be a healthy part of a meat diet. Buy these if you can find an organic farm. Our ancestors used the whole animal as food. The French, healthier than Americans, still enjoy dishes using internal organs. Buy cheese from the British Isles. They have stricter standards and ban some of our foods.

You might try wild meat or that which is organically grown. It is more expensive but since you should have only a four-ounce or six-ounce serving, it's comparable in price to a bigger, cheaper steak. Since birds make more efficient use of their feed, it would be even better if red-meat eaters could find a source of emu or ostrich meat. These birds require much less water, land and feed than cattle. My father was a hunter in Colorado and my favorite form of fowl was wild-duck. Even the breast meat was red and much more flavorful than any white-breasted chicken or turkey.

Food Pyramids that are better than the old USDA pyramid

The Oldways Preservation and Exchange Trust has four pyramids that are superior to the ones used by the USDA [these are printed with permission in the Addendum. They are based on the actual food eaten by average healthy people in four different areas: Mediterranean, Asian, Latin American and vegetarian diets. The average U.S. dieter just concentrates on food, but EXERCISE is at the base of each pyramid as the most important component. These new pyramids emphasize daily consumption of grains, fruits and vegetables but vary in the positions of oils, dairy, fish, poultry, eggs or beans and nuts. Sweets are always near the tip of the pyramid, just before red meat.

There was no mention on the pyramids for packaged junk foods. However, like the USDA pyramid that lists pasta along with bread and cereals, the Mediterranean diet includes pasta and the Asian diet lists noodles. Just as a runner can eat more carbohydrates, the people in the countries on which these diets are based get lots of exercise so they can use these simple carbohydrates.

You'll be healthier using any of these alternatives to the old USDA food pyramid that contributed to obesity because of its emphasis on grain products. Remember - the Oldways pyramids are based on the actual activity and diets of the groups studied; the first component is exercise. Foods on the lower part of the various pyramids are eaten daily. Healthy oils are used at least weekly and sweets or red meat less often. The Oldways food pyramids all report alcohol in moderation, such as red wine in a Mediterranean diet or beer in other diets.

Water in the Mediterranean, Asian, Latin American and vegetarian diets are based on what most people were drinking. On average, they drink six glasses of water daily, not eight glasses. It should depend on your size, level of activity and the temperature if you're outside. Moreover, someone on a high-protein diet needs more water to dilute the uric acid and urea in his urine.

In "The Schwarzbein Principle", Diana Schwarzbein says the USDA pyramid is doing harm

It causes people to overeat carbohydrates. She illustrates her diet idea with a square, not a pyramid, emphasizing balance. As an endocrinologist, she has been able to reverse eating disorders, type II diabetes and cardiovascular disease by getting patients away from high-carbohydrate diets that have been disturbing their metabolism and increasing the risk of heart attacks and cancer. Unlike Dr. Atkins or the Doctors Eades, she doesn't say to eat mostly protein foods and little or none with carbohydrates, such as grains or fruit. She says to eat protein, natural fat, a non-starchy vegetable and a natural carbohydrate at every meal. The carbohydrate can be a piece of fruit or a true whole-grain product. Snacks should include protein foods like cheese or nuts, never carbohydrates alone.

Besides curing glucose addictions, Dr. Schwarzbein tries to get her patients off all stimulants and most prescriptions. She says that carbohydrate eaters consume caffeine to boost their energy when too much insulin lowers their blood sugar. A balanced diet corrects this.

Paul and Patricia Bragg are early proponents of natural foods for a healthy diet

They lived in southern California and helped some Hollywood stars improve their bodies. Exercise guru Jack La Lanne used most of their diet principles. He is now over ninety and still going strong. The Braggs never recommended counting calories or grams of fat, carbohydrate, protein or fiber. They said to look at your hand. The thumb represents protein, a basic constituent of all life. It is vital to eat every day, whether you get it in meat, milk, fish, eggs, cheese or beans and nuts. Three fingers represent vegetables and fruit. The fifth represents the total of grains, fats and sugars. Therefore if 60 percent of the portions on your plate are vegetables and 20 percent is a protein source, you won't crave any manufactured foods with their processed carbohydrates and fats. Use whole-grain products along with natural fats like butter.

Meals should be more than simple nourishment for your body.

Several experts have excellent recipes in their books. Try those from the Braggs' book *Gourmet Health Recipes.* Dr. Schwarzbein has two complete recipe books. Her cookbook just for vegetarians has more than 350 recipes similar to her *The Schwarzbein Principle Cookbook* that has helped diabetics and others with metabolic diseases. *The Protein Power Life Plan,* by the doctors Eades, has menus and suggestions for feeding hungry teens when everyone in the family is busy.

The Healing Foods by Patricia Hausman and Judith Benn Hurley has many delicious natural food recipes. In addition they list conditions, from allergies to wound healing, that might be helped by eating certain foods. Their charts compare foods as good, better or best for various nutrients and fiber. People are different with somewhat different needs. One size does not fit all

Eat according to a simple system, always with natural foods

Use Braggs' idea of looking at your hand to always have a protein source, three-fifths of your meal as vegetables and some fruit and a minor portion, whole-grains and fats. Dr. Schwarzbien's diet square might be better. Each meal or snack should have protein, natural fat, a green vegetable and either a piece of fruit or whole-grain carbohydrate.

Cheese or nuts would cover both the protein and fat needs. (I can go for hours after a quick lunch of white Irish cheddar cheese on thin slices of Trader Joe's firm walnut bread with lots of lettuce or spinach leaves.) Try one of the Oldways food pyramids. The arrangement of the Latin American pyramid has less emphasis on grain products than do others.

You don't have to be obsessed with food and carry a book that lists nutrients. Get a general idea of main sources of protein, fat, fiber and carbohydrate. Then eat only real foods, not those that have been manufactured and packaged containing substances only a chemist can understand. Avoid a product with a long shelf life. If it won't support the life of an insect or a mold, it might not have the proper nutrients for human cells. Snack foods sold as energy bars might contain trans fats, fructose and other chemicals. If you need quick energy, carry a mixture of dried fruit, seeds and nuts.

Your first goal should be to improve your health. With a wide variety of natural foods, you won't be hungry for foods with empty calories. You will have more energy for moderate exercise that helps you lose fat. Getting healthy is much more important than just losing weight. Many thin people have metabolic conditions like osteoporosis as well as cancer and heart disease. Obesity, diabetes, cardiovascular disease and cancer are not inevitable as we grow older. Eating nutritious natural foods along with getting adequate exercise can prevent the disabilities of aging.

You don't have to be a fanatic. If you're not allergic or hypersensitive, a rare small serving of a rich dessert or some deep fried food won't hurt you as long as you're eating right 95 percent of the time. The total experience of eating with other people should outweigh being obsessive about your diet. Avoid extremes and aim for the Golden Mean to get maximum health.

Diet Suggestions for Your Health

- Eat three or four large servings of vegetables daily and a cup or two of salad greens.

- Eat one to three pieces of whole fruit or equivalent half-cup servings of frozen fruit. To lose weight, have one serving of fruit, low in calories like melon or high in antioxidants like berries. Juice is not an adequate substitute because it lacks fiber or bioflavonoids.

- Eat a protein food at every meal or snack. It can be from meat, fish, eggs, dairy, tofu, beans, seeds or nuts.

- Don't eat much meat. Avoid meat from factory farms.

- Get a proper balance of essential fatty acids. Get omega-3 fatty acids from a serving a day of wild salmon or other fatty, cold water fish or from walnuts, flax seed or flax oil, not other vegetable oils

- Eat wheat germ, seeds and most nuts for adequate omega-6 fatty acids. Cook with olive oil, a healthy mono-saturated oil and use it on salads or use peanut or canola oils.

- Eat butter as a stable source of energy if it's organic. I buy Irish butter.

- Be moderate with grains. Bread is beneficial if made from whole-grain and without additives. Do not eat refined carbohydrate products. Whole-grains contain minerals, a natural ratio of the B complex vitamins and both soluble and insoluble natural fiber.

- Avoid manufactured packaged foods. They often contain trans fats and high fructose corn syrup that your liver makes into the fat and LDL cholesterol that can clog your arteries.

- Avoid soft drinks because of the sugars they contain as well as phosphoric acid that can deplete your bones of calcium.

- Take time to enjoy your food and eat right 95 percent of the time. Appreciate sociable occasions even if you might have to eat a small portion of an unhealthy food.

- Aim for the Golden Mean between being a boring, obsessive ascetic and a self-indulgent or careless consumer.

  Note: Any diet must be accompanied by adequate exercise as described in later chapters.

Dietary
Supplements

Our bodies evolved by eating the plants and animals in various environments. People on a mixed diet could be healthy in most parts of the world. When they restricted their diets to a few items, they got deficiency diseases.

Asians who ate mostly white rice without the husk and germ got beriberi. Poor southerners in the U.S. who subsisted on corn and salt pork got pellagra. Sailors who had no fresh foods for months got scurvy, characterized by bleeding gums and sore joints. These and other diseases affecting skin, eyes, muscles, bones, joints, the intestinal tract and the nervous system were all caused by the lack of one or more vitamins in their diet.

The Food and Drug Administration recommends minimum amounts to prevent deficiency diseases

The basic food groups should have had enough vitamins. Manufacturers stripped foods of many nutrients to get products that could be packaged and sold for a higher price. The Irish received proteins, vitamins and minerals as well as starches from boiled potatoes, but potato chips have nothing but calories. Many breakfast cereals have few of the nutrients of the original whole-grains. You can't make up for a junk food diet by taking vitamins. This might prevent deficiency diseases but you need natural whole foods for optimum health.

Ideal doses of vitamins, minerals or other supplements can depend on age and special circumstances

The book *Nutraceuticals: The Complete Encyclopedia of Supple-*

ments, Herbs, Vitamins and Healing Foods by Arthur Roberts covers a range of situations, mentioning special needs such as pregnancy. One size does not fit all. Other special circumstances might be travel to a country with environmental pollution such as Russia or China; another is before and after surgery. In general, as long as you're eating a healthy diet, it's better to take a smaller dose of a supplement rather than too much, especially in the case of minerals and the fat-soluble vitamins.

Minerals are important substances. Most are contained within our food but can be lost if cooking water is discarded. In order to get enough of others, we must take them in pill form.

Antioxidants are contained in foods or made within our own cells to use as needed.

Nutraceuticals are special substances from herbs or other sources that act as pharmaceuticals to relieve symptoms or help the body heal itself and cure a disease.

14-1 Vitamins

Vitamins are necessary but do you know what they are or what they do? You have heard that vitamin A is good for the eyes, the various B vitamins are good for the nerves and skin and help the liver metabolize alcohol, that vitamin C prevents scurvy and vitamin D helps build strong bones. We now know that vitamin E helps the cardiovascular system and that vitamin K helps the blood to clot.

Most vitamins must be accompanied by the essential amino acids and essential fatty acids of a good balanced diet. If you eat junk food, even high potency vitamins won't keep you healthy.

Vitamins are small but complex molecules that humans mostly get in their food

Vitamin D can also be made in the body by sunlight striking the skin. Vitamin B-12, cyancobalamin, isn't contained in food at all. If a person eats even a small amount of eggs, milk or meat, the bacteria in his colon use these animal proteins to make vitamin B-12. This vitamin helps make healthy red blood cells and healthy nerves. Only a strict vegan-type vegetarian would need to take this vitamin. Forty years ago it was only given by injection. Many multivitamin pills now contain B-12, but it is best taken as a small tablet dissolved under your tongue. That way it is absorbcd dirclass into small blood vessels there and can't be changed. Vitamin K that promotes normal clotting is also made by intestinal bacteria.

Many vitamins act as co-enzymes (co-factors of enzymes) and others are antioxidants

In chemical reactions inside the cells of the human body, the vitamin, as a co-enzyme, guides the substances in a chemical reaction so they attach to a certain place on the enzyme, a large protein molecule. Together they help to form a product quickly and efficiently. The added function of some vitamins such as A, C, and E as antioxidants was discovered later. In this role they protect cells from the action of activated oxygen or free radicals generated by chemical reactions within cells.

Linus Pauling Ph.D., made a name in popular literature by advocating very large amounts of vitamin C, also known as ascorbic acid. His rationale was that unlike most animals, man and the higher apes can't make ascorbic acid and must get it from food. He said that since the gorilla is a vegetarian and gets lots of ascorbic acid from green plants, humans should take many grams of it in pill form to be comparable. Pauling received a Nobel Prize in chemistry on the nature of the hydrogen bond and a later Nobel Peace Prize.

However, he didn't go far enough in his study of comparative physiology. Humans are more like chimpanzees, since we are both omnivores. Unlike the gorilla, our blood contains a significant amount of uric acid. This is a molecule composed of two different rings of carbon atoms. It has several double bonds so acts as an antioxidant. However, it can't protect the body from scurvy as does vitamin C. Stay healthy by taking a moderate amount of vitamin C daily, 100 mg to 500 mg. This can be increased to 1 or 2 grams to ward off a cold then gradually decreased back to a normal dose. If you stop taking it abruptly, you might get symptoms of deficiency such as bleeding gums. The book *Nutraceuticals* warns that taking more than 1,000 mg a day can *increase* oxidative damage from free radicals instead of protecting against it.

Some people take many supplements that aren't necessary and might have side effects

One friend almost had a panic attack when he forgot to bring his vitamins and many herbal pills on a weekend excursion. I could only reassure him that some of the substances have been retained in his body fat to use as needed. Others might enhance certain reactions, but his cells don't come to a screeching halt without them.

The book *Nutritional Pharmacology*, edited by Gene Spiller, tells of many instances when a person damaged his body by taking too many supplements. This is especially true of minerals and the fat-soluble vitamins A, D, and E. There can be side effects of too-high doses even of water-soluble vitamin C. In doses over 1,000 mg., it can cause diarrhea and can be a bladder irritant in doses over 500 mg. for some people. This is okay if you're taking large amounts to ward off a cold and drinking more fluids anyway. Perhaps taking too much vitamin C is one of the causes of a rising increase in the numbers of people of all ages with urinary urgency.

Most of the B vitamins are co-enzymes in multiple reactions within the cells. The B complex includes thiamin, riboflavin, niacin, pantothenic acid, pyridoxine and biotin. Any deficiency can produce a variety of signs. These can range from decreased energy to scaly or abnormally red skin to gastro-intestinal distress to what was called a nervous breakdown.

Mabel noticed changes in the behavior of her roommate Betty, who had been working day and night trying to finish her Ph.D thesis. She screamed when anyone tried to talk with her and never seemed to eat or sleep. She never went outdoors, but her skin was a bright pink. One night Mabel heard her sobbing in the bathroom saying that demons were giving her headaches and she couldn't go on. Mabel, a nutritionist, thought she might be deficient in niacin and other B vitamins. She gave her a good multivitamin pill, then warm milk with added wheat germ and brewer's yeast. A good diet with high doses of B vitamins helped Betty get back to normal as she postponed her scheduled graduation. According to Mabel's description, Betty had the beginning of the classic three "D's" of pellagra: a sunburn-like dermatitis, diarrhea and dementia.

High doses of niacin have been used for many years to decrease cholesterol levels. However, most patients don't like the itchy flush. Most multivitamin tablets use a derivative of niacin called nicotinamide that doesn't cause flushing. It doesn't help lower cholesterol but is still good for other functions of vitamin B-3, like keeping skin and nerves healthy and helping to prevent pellagra.

The B vitamin, biotin, is widespread in foods and some is made by intestinal bacteria. No one who isn't starving should be deficient. But some health conscious persons with little time for breakfast have suffered from a lack of biotin, getting symptoms such as itchy dry skin and hair loss. They would make a smoothie with fruit and milk and throw in a raw egg. The raw egg white contains avidin, a protein that hooks on to the biotin in other foods and makes it unavailable. (Another reason not to eat raw eggs is they might have salmonella bacteria.)

A recent advertisement for a multiple vitamin said that it contains extra biotin for people on an Atkins diet. This is a gimmick. Biotin is a coenzyme for reactions in carbohydrate and fat metabolism but in excess causes the liver to produce too much fat and cholesterol and also interfere with other B vitamins. Stay with natural high sources like liver, peanuts, dried peas, wheat germ or mushrooms and you won't get too much.

Many high potency multivitamins have equally high amounts of each of the B vitamins

In the past, many physicians have said, "You're just wasting your money and producing expensive urine." In the wrong proportion, the use of some B vitamins interferes with the action of others. Don't count on the excretion of the excess. Wheat germ and brewers yeast are a good source of all the B vitamins that I have relied on for many years. Add a couple spoonfuls of each to cereals or salads.

After a party, before going to bed, one friend always has a tablespoonful of brewer's yeast in water to counteract the extra alcohol he drank. Several years ago, someone suggested a law for manufacturers to add B vitamins to distilled spirits to protect the livers of the drinkers. Distillers opposed this as unwarranted regulation and teetotalers didn't like the idea of safer consumption of "demon rum." People who drink home brew always get a little of the yeast that settles to the bottom of the beer bottle as sediment. However this is filtered off and removed in commercial beers. Heavy drinkers of distilled spirits should take thiamine to protect their livers. Even a mild deficiency of thiamine can cause numbness and tingling of the legs.

Vitamin B-12 must always be in addition to a diet with enough folic acid. Both are necessary in the building of red blood cells and to prevent tingling and numbness in the nerves. As mentioned before, vitamin B-6, pyridoxine, is necessary with vitamin B-12 and folic acid to prevent the damage of homocysteine on blood vessels. A mixed diet with plenty of fruits and raw green vegetables as well as some meat should provide all of these nutrients.

The need for Vitamin D

Rickets is a bone disease caused by a lack of vitamin D. During the Industrial Revolution, coal smoke blocked out the sun's rays so a person's skin cells couldn't make vitamin D. This vitamin helps in bone formation, so bow-legs and other signs of rickets were common. Cod liver oil was one of the first supplements introduced because it contained vitamin D and cured rickets, but children didn't like the fishy taste. Around the 1930s, milk was treated with ultra-violet light to change ergosterol into active vitamin D which stayed in the cream. Milk was then homogenized so cream no longer rose to the top for adults to use in coffee. Fat with its vitamin D was in tiny droplets throughout the milk, so was available to all who drank it.

This worked well until consumers became afraid of fat. Adults started drinking skim milk and often gave it to their children. They didn't even eat butter. Now both adults and children have to take vitamin tablets for the missing vitamin D and also a lack of vitamin A in skim milk. Get your vitamin D in irradiated whole milk. Or form it naturally by getting into direct sunlight without sunscreen for three 15-minute periods per week. This is not enough to cause damage or promote skin cancer in the average person.

Vitamins A, D, and E are the fat-soluble vitamins and can remain in your body fat for weeks

It isn't necessary to take them every day. They are best absorbed when taken with a meal that contains fat.

Steve's doctor told him he was getting calcium deposits in his muscles and to stop taking calcium pills. The real problem might have been his getting too much vitamin D along with extra vitamins A and E. More is not better. These fat-soluble vitamins can increase each other's action. They must have caused too much calcium to stay in his system. Too much of any of these fat-soluble vitamins can cause trouble.

Excess vitamin A can cause liver damage or worse. Even natural sources might contain too much. Explorers in the Arctic found that polar bear liver acted like a poison because of the very high concentration of vitamin A. Most multiple vitamin tablets now have it in the safer form of beta-carotene. It's better to get beta-carotene and related compounds in orange vegetables like yams, carrots and squash. The body then makes it into vitamin A.

Since people who ate carrots or other orange foods were less susceptible to cancer, a study in Finland was done several years ago to see if male smokers could be protected by taking vitamin A or beta-carotene. Many smokers still died of lung cancer as reported in the *New England Journal of Medicine* 330:1029-1035,

1994 by Dr. O.P. Heinonen and others.

In a similar study by the National Cancer Institute called CARET (Carotene and Retinol Efficacy Trial) of 18,000 smokers, matched groups received 25,000 units of vitamin A, 30 mg. of beta-carotene, both or none. The experiment was terminated when the men taking either of the supplements died of lung cancer at a higher rate than other smokers. There was no logical explanation, but a lot of controversy.

Maybe these synthetic substances upset the basic chemistry of the lung tissue. What the studies showed is that no pill overcomes the deleterious effects of smoking. Whole foods are better than pills because they contain other active ingredients, sometimes in trace amounts.

Supplement your healthy diet with a minimal dose multivitamin pill. It should have balanced values of B vitamins. An excess of even the water-soluble B vitamins and vitamin C might not be harmless. *Nutritional Pharmacology* edited by Gene Spiller, related many cases of individual adverse reactions to high doses of some vitamins and minerals. High amounts of vitamins can't compensate for a junk food diet. A diet of processed foods and soft drinks is deficient, even if some of the vitamins lost during manufacture are added back. Natural foods give optimal doses. Everyone needs the essential amino acids and essential fatty acids contained in meat, fish and eggs or in soy products, seeds and nuts. Besides vitamins, they also need the myriad antioxidants and minerals in fruits and vegetables.

14-2 Minerals

Iron is one of the most important minerals in your body

In normal people, iron enters the blood stream as ferritin. This is carried to the liver or bone marrow to make hemoglobin, a carrier of the oxygen necessary for life. Iron is also in red muscle cells as myoglobin and is in the enzymes of the cytochrome system. Cytochromes are the final link between metabolic processes and molecular oxygen. This vital enzyme system is inactivated by cyanide and carbon monoxide as well as some insecticides. Iron is best obtained from food so you won't get too much. Good sources are liver, heart, red meat, egg yolks, raisins and soybeans.

Iron in your diet might not be used properly by your body

Iron plus some vitamins is added to baked goods and cereals. This isn't good for some people. You can get too much iron into your blood stream if your body reacts against the lectins in wheat and other grains. Intestinal cells injured by lectins don't allow the cells in the intestinal villi to sequester excess iron. In the normal person, iron not needed by the body collects in special cells sloughed off every few days along with other cells in the small intestine.

Extra iron in pill form can cause black stools from iron sulfide formed by normal intestinal bacteria. However, black tarry stools unrelated to extra iron indicate intestinal bleeding that should be checked by your physician. Any man with low hemoglobin is probably losing blood from his stomach or intestines. This might indicate cancer or bleeding caused by drugs like aspirin or ibuprofen.

Ferritin iron can collect in large amounts in persons with hemochromatosis. This is a hereditary disease that damages the heart, liver and other organs. The Doctors Eades in their book *The Protein Power Life Plan* say that a growing number of persons even without this genetic disorder might be collecting excess iron in their bodies. To prevent this iron from being deposited in vital organs, the Eades suggest regularly donating blood. If people over sixty don't feel energetic, it usually is not because of "tired blood" that needs a shot of iron.

Anemia is much more wide-spread than hemachromatosis

The 2001 book *Nutraceuticals* says that anemia is still common despite laws to add iron to breads and cereals. Many women continue being anemic while consuming this added iron. It might not be absorbed because of the phytates in grain products or because of tannins in tea. You can absorb more iron by taking vitamin C with your iron pill. Even this might not increase your hemoglobin.

A few years ago, I found out that my hemoglobin was only 12.6 gm. This explained why my pulse rate got very high when I followed younger hikers up a steep path at 5,000 feet. I didn't expect the 14.6 gm. I had when I lived in Colorado, but I shouldn't be borderline anemic. A year of daily vitamin pills with 15 mg. iron did not raise my hemoglobin. I continued weekly hikes but started taking a 10 mg. capsule of DHEA (dehydroepiandrosterone), along with a multivitamin with only 5 mg. iron. After several months, my hemoglobin value increased to 13.2 gm.

DHEA is a pre-hormone that the body can make into either androgens or estrogens. It can be dangerous. Some body builders have damaged their livers with very high doses. This supplement should be monitored. A good philosophy with any supplement is to take the smallest amount that gives a desired result. I doubt that a higher dose of DHEA would raise my hemoglobin more. Only living for several months at a high altitude would do this. Men are lucky, since their testosterone helps their blood cells make hemoglobin from the iron in their diet.

You never outgrow your need for calcium

Despite the ads that say "You never outgrow your need for milk," many adults can't drink it because of lactose intolerance, the inability to use milk sugar. They are told to take one to two grams of calcium in pill form every day. Swallowing a pill doesn't mean it will be absorbed. One doctor was mystified by oblong objects he saw in the x-ray of the intestines of a patient. They were calcium pills that hadn't dissolved.

Advertisers and health maintenance organizations advise patients to get calcium by chewing Tums, Rolaids or a similar antacid. Most of these have added sugar and flavor. Such a cloying candy mint is bad for teeth and gums. I prefer an easily chewed wafer with a clean chalky taste. Formerly, I could buy calcium carbonate powder. Instead of dissolving it in juice or soup, I put a small amount on the end of a spoon. This dissolved instantly in my saliva and was easily washed down with water.

Calcium must be balanced with the proper amounts of magnesium and phosphorus

This can help prevent osteoporosis. There is always a certain amount of calcium as well as other minerals in your blood stream. Even though your bones look solid, some calcium ions come out of your bones every day and new calcium is deposited where needed, as long as you have the proper amounts of phosphorus and magnesium in your diet in balance with calcium. Phosphorus from a high meat diet can draw calcium out of the bones to be excreted. Strict vegetarians, known as vegans, have been misled that eggs and cheese might also cause osteoporosis. In reality, cheese has about nine parts calcium to seven parts phosphorus; eggs have a ratio of about 1 to 2. Meat, however, has 10 to 20 times more phosphorus than calcium. Those who stay on a high-meat Atkins diet can lose a lot of calcium.

The phosphates in many soft drinks also remove calcium from your bones and cause its excretion. Teenagers who should be strengthening their bones with dairy products instead are thinning them by substituting sweet carbonated drinks for milk. Children are now drinking more soft drinks than milk and are not building strong bones. Many women in their thirties already have thinner bones, leading to osteoporosis at menopause and then brittle broken bones in old age.

Caffeine in coffee and other beverages bind calcium and make it unavailable. Caffeine-free diet soft drinks aren't harmless either, since they contain phosphoric acid that causes calcium loss. When you're pregnant, the growing baby takes calcium. You need extra calcium to prevent osteoporosis. In the nineteenth century, they said that a woman loses a tooth with every pregnancy.

Bones need the stimulation of exercise or weight-bearing to gain or retain calcium

You can't keep your bones from losing calcium just by taking calcium even when balanced with enough magnesium and adequate vitamin D. If you're not putting stress on your skeleton, the added calcium will not be absorbed. I found this out in my twenties when I was in medical school. I had fallen off a glacier, breaking both lower leg bones on the right. The tibia had to be fastened together with screws and the fibula was so shattered, it was ignored. I was put into a cast from hip to toes. Conventional treatment was to immobilize both the knee joint and the ankle joint. I was given a pair of crutches but told not to put any weight on the foot. This precaution was valid at first to prevent forming cartilage instead of bone between the broken pieces.

But in later X-rays, the break wasn't healing and the shin bone was becoming less dense, indicating loss of calcium. Vitamin D and increased milk didn't stop this loss or aid in calcification of the broken bone.

I then put weight-bearing stress on the bones of the broken leg. I rested the foot of my cast on my bathroom scales and transferred a measured amount of weight to it. I increased it two or three pounds a day. By the end of the month, there was no more fading away of the leg bones in the x-ray. As I continued to increase the amount of weight I put on the leg, each x-ray looked better. By the end of the seventh month, I went to a knee-high walking cast. At this point a friend took me dancing.

The following year, more orthopedists were putting a long rod through a broken leg bone to stabilize it inside the cast and telling patients they could put weight on the foot after several days. A friend with this treatment was out of his cast in less than four months. This emphasizes the point that your bones can use and keep calcium only if stressed by weight bearing. Astronauts in space have a similar problem. They must do resistance exercises to keep their bones from losing calcium to be excreted in the urine.

You need a balanced diet with adequate calories to have strong bones

A thin woman who subsists on salads might not be aware that the gradual loss of calcium from her bones or a decrease in muscle mass makes her less healthy than the woman of normal weight. Even before age 60 she'll start noticing problems. A thin friend is now getting a hunched back as calcium in her spine has been depleted. During testing at a recent health fair, I noticed that a couple of older obese women had bone density values about 115 percent greater than a normal 26-year old. Besides the stimulation of added weight, their fat cells make more estrogen. Two thin women had values under 70 percent. My bone density was 139 percent of a 26-year-old woman.

Endocrinologist Dr. Schwarzbein tells her patients that bones need protein for a matrix on which calcium salts are deposited. Dietary fat and cholesterol are also necessary to make the sex hormones that help in bone formation. Some women joggers have found that a low-fat, high-carbohydrate diet and exercising too much have made their bones as thin and brittle as those of an old crone, despite their taking calcium pills. The author of *The Schwarzbein Principle* says that osteoporosis can be reversed with a balanced diet containing plenty of calcium-rich foods, along with moderate exercise. Her patients avoid alcohol, caffeine and anti-inflammatory drugs. She advocates hormone replacement in menopause. Estrogen does help the bones stay strong.

Since caffeine can combine with calcium in your diet and make some of it unavailable, you might want to take your calcium at a different time than with your morning coffee. On the other hand, the calcium-bound caffeine might prevent the unwanted nervousness of too much stimulation. Try it and see the timing that works best for you. The European habit of adding a third hot milk to their morning cup of strong coffee moderates the effect of caffeine.

You need a pure source of calcium and magnesium

Years ago in England, the bones of horses were used to make bone meal. Many horses pulled delivery wagons and were exposed to the exhaust of automobiles using leaded gasoline. Thus a person got lead in his bone meal along with the needed calcium and magnesium. Mined mineral dolomite was then taken for its calcium and magnesium until analysis showed traces of arsenic. Oyster shell calcium is probably all right. You don't need expensive ground-up coral from Okinawa, despite the miracles attributed to it. Some tablets with both calcium and magnesium are hard to chew and also include zinc. If the multivitamin, multimineral supplement you're taking already has 15 mg. zinc, you don't need more of that mineral. However, you never outgrow your need for both calcium and magnesium.

Magnesium, besides its role in strong bones and teeth, is important in cell metabolism

Magnesium is a cofactor within the cells in hundreds of enzymatic reactions. It can block calcium ions from getting into cells where they aren't needed. When given intravenously, it can decrease high blood pressure and has been used for decades in pregnant women with toxemia. Now doctors in emergency rooms give magnesium for heart attacks, acute asthma or in intensive care emergencies.

Since high insulin causes the kidneys to excrete magnesium, The Doctors Eades use it for patients with all the conditions associated with increased insulin, including type II diabetes, high blood pressure, heart disease, obesity, high cholesterol and high triglycerides. They speculate that some patients have low magnesium inside their cells even when serum levels are normal. These include chronic fatigue syndrome, migraines, asthma and other allergies, seizures and panic reactions.

How many patients could stop taking expensive medications if their intracellular magnesium were brought back to normal? If indeed more than 70 percent of Americans aren't getting enough magnesium in their diets, maybe they can be cured by this inexpensive mineral. Wouldn't it be worth trying first?

Magnesium ions have a position in chlorophyll like that of iron in hemoglobin. You would need to eat a lot of leafy green plants to get enough. Cows secrete both magnesium and calcium in their milk. However, it's the wrong ratio for humans.

In the days of the family farm, magnesium was concentrated in grains. Now that chemical fertilizers add only phosphorus, potassium and nitrates, there's not much magnesium or other minerals in most grains. Nuts, beans, peas and other legumes contain some magnesium, as does some hard well water. Most U.S. bottled waters don't have many minerals. Most people should take 200 to 400 mg. of magnesium per day. It is best absorbed as the citrate or malate. Even in less expensive pills combining calcium, magnesium and zinc, it is one supplement we all need for optimum health. Taken at night it helps promote sleep. Don't shun magnesium just because a much higher dose is used for constipation as "Milk of Magnesia".

Potassium and sodium are both needed by your body

Potassium is contained in all fruit and vegetables. You get it and most other minerals in your diet from fruit and vegetables, as long as you use the cooking water that contains the minerals. You need some salt so don't cut it out, just cut back. We all need about a fourth of the 2.1 grams of sodium in a teaspoon of salt. Some sodium is important to regulate fluids in the blood and body tissues. Similarly, potassium controls fluids within our cells. We usually get the necessary 2 grams of potassium per day since it exists in all plant and animal cells. But with activities that make you perspire a lot, you need to replenish both sodium and potassium.

In the jungles of Suriname, the rice and vegetables were highly salted to help us cope with the heat. We noticed swelling of our ankles as the excess sodium made our tissues retain water. One person felt weak, perhaps from potassium loss, but felt normal after drinking fruit juice.

Some athletes take potassium pills after exercise in the heat to treat their severe muscle cramps. That can be dangerous. Excess potassium can cause an abnormal rhythm of the heart and interfere with muscle contraction. A balanced sports drink would be better. Too much salt (sodium chloride) is less dangerous. It does not cause high blood pressure in people with normal kidneys.

Zinc is a co-factor in many enzymatic reactions

It is necessary for growth, immunity, wound healing, sexual development and reproduction. The best food sources are oysters, liver, meat, nuts and wheat germ. People with certain skin diseases may need twice the recommended 15 mg. per day. Some people think that sucking zinc lozenges will shorten the duration of a cold. It might be harmful if you're not careful. Dr. Jeff Victoroff in *Saving Your Brain* says that too much zinc can damage cells in the nervous system. Long-term use of high amounts can also damage your immune system.

Copper can act as a co-factor in the same metabolic reactions that need zinc

It promotes the healing of wounds and burns. It also helps the body to use iron, make collagen in connective tissue and the myelin around nerves. Good sources are oysters and shellfish, blackstrap molasses, seeds, nuts, wheat germ, soybeans, avocados and green olives. Most people don't need an added dose of 1.5 to 3 mg. in a pill. However, some women with osteoporosis and some men with high LDL cholesterol have quite low levels of copper and should get more.

Dr. Michael Lesser in *The Brain Chemistry Diet* says that the ratio of zinc and copper can affect the brain and a person's behavior. Relatively too much copper can cause agitation or rage. If the level is too low, you can become lethargic or depressed. Stress often raises copper and lowers zinc in the body. If you get your water from copper pipes, you don't need extra in a pill. You can lower copper levels by eating garlic, onions or radishes daily.

You need tiny amounts of manganese, fluoride, iodine, molybdenum, chromium and selenium

Trace amounts are in micrograms rather than the milligrams of major minerals. (A microgram is a millionth of a gram, while a milligram is a thousandth of a gram.)

Manganese is a mineral necessary for enzymatic reactions

It helps insulin in the metabolism of carbohydrates and synthesis of cholesterol. It works with vitamin K to help in clotting of blood and healing of wounds. Get it in rice and other wholegrains, soybeans and other legumes.

Fluoride helps in the hardening of bones and teeth

You can get your tiny daily requirement in dried seaweed, tea and canned sardines. Whether it should be in everyone's drinking water is still controversial. Some cities no longer add it, even the very low amount of 1-2 parts per billion.

Iodine needed by a normal adult for thyroid function is 150 micrograms a day

The thyroid gland controls metabolism and how all cells use oxygen. Eating too much kale or cabbage can block its absorption. Certain peoples in central Europe where the soil is deficient in iodine might not get enough. If they also eat too much cabbage, they suffer the thick skin and low metabolism of hypothyroidism. Most people get iodine in iodized salt. It's also in kelp and seafood.

Molybdenum at 75 to 250 micrograms helps in the metabolism of carbohydrate, fat and protein

It also helps control uric acid from the purine breakdown products of nucleic acids. This helps to prevent gout. Good sources are beans, wheat germ, eggs, organ meats and leafy vegetables.

Chromium at 50-100 micrograms is necessary for insulin to metabolize glucose

It also helps in the use of proteins and fats and protects DNA and RNA. When there's not enough chromium, blood sugar increases. The blood level of LDL cholesterol rises and HDL cholesterol falls, setting a person up for coronary artery disease. It may or may not increase muscle mass as less fat is formed. Best sources are liver, brewer's yeast, whole-grains, nuts, and cheese.

Selenium is part of an enzyme, glutathione peroxidase that protects DNA from free radicals

It helps vitamin E prevent the oxidation of fats and can help prevent cataracts. Vitamin E with selenium might also prevent certain cancers and help the heart by maintaining ubiquinone (coenzyme Q-10) in body tissues. If the soil has enough selenium, the needed 50 micrograms can come from wheat germ, legumes, pork, lamb, sea food, brewer's yeast or black-strap molasses.

Get the right amount of minerals for good health, not too much

Sign of an overdose of any minor mineral are nausea and vomiting. Most adults should take added calcium, 500 to 1000 mg. in addition to that in cheese and soy products. Since milk products don't have enough magnesium, take an extra 200 to 400 mg. Minimum doses of a multiple vitamin and mineral tablet probably will provide enough of other minerals except in unusual circumstances. A person at risk of heart disease needs extra selenium. Diabetics need extra chromium to help stabilize their insulin and increase their body's sensitivity to it. Athletes might need some extra potassium after excessive perspiration. Some people need added zinc or copper.

14-3 Antioxidants

Antioxidants act within body cells to protect them from oxidative damage. They counteract the harmful effects of singlet oxygen (O-) hydroxyl (OH-) or free radicals.

These all try to pass on a free electron or gain another one to form a more stable compound. After a series of complex reactions, stable atoms such as water or carbon dioxide are formed and energy is produced. Meanwhile, antioxidants react with the hyperactive oxygen or other rogue molecules. These are then passed on to another antioxidant and then another. The end result is that without the antioxidant system, reactive atoms or molecules could damage your DNA or cause changes in enzymes necessary for cell metabolism. It's like throwing a monkey wrench into a fine machine. Without antioxidants, reactive molecules could also cause stiffening of cell membranes so reactants can't get through as well.

An antioxidant network within your cells is described by Dr. Lester Packer in his book *The Antioxidant Miracle.* In a healthy body, each antioxidant is continually regenerated by another one and recycled many times. Vitamin E is the master chemical that renews vitamin C, which regenerates glutathione, which renews lipoic acid, thereby renewing coenzyme Q-10 (ubiqui-none). Glutathione, lipoic acid and coenzyme Q-10 are all made in your body from amino acids. Lipoic acid is of special impor-tance, since it can dissolve either in the fat of cell membranes or the liquids inside the cells. It can even take over when vitamin E is low. Packer calls lipoic acid a "superman molecule," since very large doses have saved persons from radiation exposure, hepatitis C and even amanita mushroom poisoning.

Vitamin E is one of the most important antioxidants

This fat-soluble vitamin is carried in the blood by globules of fatty proteins. At one part per thousand, it protects the associ-ated fat and cholesterol from oxidation. It gets into cells by dis-solving in their fatty membranes. By preventing fat peroxides from forming, it helps prevent cellular aging. Vitamin E has other properties: enhance the immune system, help the body fight cancer, decrease the inflammation of arthritis, slow down Alzheimer's disease and help prevent cataracts. Packer says related molecules called tocotrienols can unclog the carotid arteries leading to the brain and prevent certain strokes.

In "The Wrinkle Cure", Nicholas Perricone says lipoic acid can penetrate skin cells

Since it dissolves in either water or fat, it combats the free radicals that act on the skin as well as those inside the body. It helps heal sunburn damage from ultra-violet rays. In deeper cells, a high blood sugar can cause cross-linkages in body pro-teins making them less flexible. In the skin, this produces wrin-kles as both the collagen and the blood vessels become stiff. Perricone says that lipoic acid, along with ascorbyl palmitate and DMAE (di-methyl amino ethanol), can reverse these effects if applied to the skin. It must be accompanied by a low-sugar diet containing adequate protein, essential fatty acids, supple-mental vitamins E and C and oral lipoic acid.

Ubiquinone (coenzyme Q-10) is an important fat-soluble antioxidant

It recycles vitamin E within your cells. It is vital for the energy cycle in all your cells. Your body makes it on a healthy diet. As you get older, be sure to eat salmon, liver and other organ meats. Many cardiac patients and diabetics are now being given statin-type drugs to get the liver to stop making LDL cholesterol. Since coenzyme Q-10 is also depleted by these statin drugs, it should be taken along with them to protect the liver and other organs. If your doctor hasn't suggested it with your cholesterol-lowering drug, hurry to a health food store to get coenzyme Q-10 (ubiquinone). It is necessary for all your cells and might protect you from muscle damage or other harmful effects of statins.

The flavonoids or bioflavonoids are important antioxidants made by plants

They are often brightly colored compounds as in berries, cherries, grapes, tomatoes, yellow and orange vegetables and green tea. Most are polyphenols that help recycle vitamins C and E and scavenge free radicals. They protect the heart by preventing the oxidation of LDL cholesterol and prevent clots in blood vessels. They also help regulate nitric acid, allowing vessels to expand and reduce high blood pressure. Some studies suggest they can improve the blood supply to the brain, so are useful in attention deficit disorder. This is a reason for children to eat colored berries, not shun them as suggested in early works by Dr. Ben Feingold.

Most flavonoids are best when consumed in raw fruits and vegetables. However, the lycopenes in tomatoes become available only by cooking. Studies show that people who eat the most bioflavonoids had the lowest risk of cancer and heart disease. Flavonoids prevent inflammation in blood vessels and other tissues, protect DNA from mutation, fight viruses and enhance the immune system. These are important reasons to eat plenty of fruits and vegetables.

The essential omega-3 and omega-6 fatty acids are best consumed in foods. You can get the omega-3 linolenic acid from walnuts, flax seeds or fatty fish like salmon and sardines. Do not discard the skin, as this contains most of these nutrients. Flax oil capsules are a good source of more linolenic acid. Sardines in olive oil are superior to those packed in water. Soy oil, however, has both linolenic and linoleic acids. Most Americans get too much of this omega-6 linoleic acid already. Most plant oils contain several fatty acids even if one predominates. Many even have a small amount of a saturated fatty acid. Evening primrose oil contains some linoleic, an omega-6 fatty acid along with gamma linolenic acid, an omega-3 fatty acid.

People on restricted diets often need more supplements

Vegan vegetarians have to take vitamin B-12 in pill form and possibly more supplements to compensate for a diet without even milk cheese or eggs. Meat eaters who have nothing but boneless, skinless chicken breasts can be deficient in iron. Even other muscle meats can lack the nutritious substances from the internal organs of animals. Liver is one of the best sources of all the B complex vitamins. As mentioned before, a healthy aspect of the French diet is the fact they eat kidneys, liver, sweet-breads (thymus gland, high in RNA) and snails. They raise small animals such as rabbits or a few larger animals that obtain more nutrients from greenery than do our factory-fed chickens, pigs or cattle.

Many substances necessary for metabolism are made by your body. Most are made and used within your cells as long as you're on a healthy diet that includes some animal products. These chemicals include ubiquinone, DHEA, carnitine, coenzyme Q-10, MSM (methylsulfonyl methane), DMSO (dimethyl sulfoxide) and glutathione. Sulfur containing supplements DMSO and MSM aren't necessary if you get enough milk, meat and broccoli for your body to make them. A healthy body makes necessary glucosamine and chondroitin for healthy cartilage.

Supplement sellers often tout specific ones to body builders and to aging adults. However, almost without exception, these chemicals are made by one's own healthy body on a nutritious diet with adequate exercise. They don't have to be taken in pill form or injected. Glutathione, said to be a super-antioxidant, is a combination of the amino acids glutamine, cysteine, and glycine. Taking it in pill form is a waste of money, since it just breaks down into those amino acids in your digestive tract. Your body cells can make all the glutathione you need from a diet of high quality proteins.

Lecithin contains choline. Half-informed sources say to take lecithin to increase the neurotransmitter acetyl-choline in your brain. Since it can't pass out of the blood vessels into the brain, lecithin either in pills or foods like soy or egg yolks won't make you smarter or improve reaction time. Dr Jeff Victoroff in *Save Your Brain* tells of failed attempts to arrest either Alzheimer's disease or senile dementia with massive doses of lecithin.

Medical Journalist Jean Carper distills the opinions of 14 experts in her book "Stop Aging Now"_

She says they agree that many of the diseases and effects of aging are caused by free radicals. This theory was first advanced by Dr. Denham Harman in the 1950s, when he was studying the effects of radiation on cells. Free radicals can come from the environment but most are formed in reactions within your cells. These can be counteracted by antioxidants that combine with these very active molecules and keep them from attacking vital chemicals inside and outside the cells.

Carper found that most of these 14 doctors she interviewed took 400 units of vitamin E each day to protect their cardiovascular systems from free radicals. Their favorite mineral is selenium. It is a co-factor for enzymes in the heart and enhances vitamin E. [In November, 2004, the media reported even moderately high doses of vitamin E have caused harm in some people. More studies are necessary. As mentioned earlier it's better to take small rather than large doses of supplements.]

Only Linus Pauling advised using 3,200 to 12,000 mg. of vitamin C (ascorbic acid) per day. Most suggested 250 to 500 mg. of this potent antioxidant. Dr. Andrew Weil used to take 1-2 gm. of ascorbic acid a day, but now advocates 500 mg or less. All these values are higher than the 30 to 60 mg. necessary to prevent scurvy.

A third of the men also take 25,000 units of beta-carotene or the equivalent of vitamin A. They have individual favorites among other supplements. These include vitamins B-6 and B-12, calcium, carnitine, chromium, coenzyme Q-10, folic acid, garlic, gingko, glutathione, magnesium and a multivitamin multimineral tablet. Carper didn't quote any women, but with half the amounts of the antioxidants taken by the men, they might slow down the aging process

Antioxidants, vitamins and minerals plus a healthy diet can prevent many of the effects of aging

As various supplements were discovered and synthesized, they were put into pills and capsules. These were to compensate for a diet of manufactured foods containing sugar, white flour and other "empty calories." The supplements helped prevent some deficiencies, but meanwhile, conditions such as constipation and heartburn increased.

You might have to take some supplements as your natural chemicals can decline with age. First, improve your diet, then exercise more to help your body increase cellular chemicals naturally. You can prevent debilitating aging. It is most important to stay on a healthy natural diet.

Future chapters explain how to get enough exercise but not too much. Other chapters emphasize the mind-body connection and the importance of interactions with other people.

14-4 Nutraceuticals

A nutraceutical is an herbal substance that doesn't need a doctor's prescription. It acts like a pharmaceutical in relieving symptoms.

It often helps the body heal itself. With the high cost of prescription drugs, more people are using herbs or other supplements and also ancient procedures like acupuncture. Some herbs have proven effective over the centuries, even if their mechanisms of action are still unknown. Some herbal remedies can keep you away from prescription drugs. They can promote a longer, healthier life as well as remove the symptoms of a disease. Besides vitamins and minerals, *Nutraceuticals,* a guide book by the American Nutraceutical Association, lists 96 separate herbs or other botanicals plus 44 nutraceutical supplements derived from or contained in various plant or animal sources.

Western scientists isolate the active chemical in any substance with healing properties

Herbalists are willing to use them as teas or extracts to relieve suffering. Medical students know the story of Dr. William Withering, who in 1775 followed a so-called witch to see what herbs she collected that healed people when his medicines were ineffective. He used a scientific method by trying the herbs one at a time. He found that only the leaves of the fox-glove *(Digitalis purpura)* relieved ankle swelling and lung congestion by strengthening the action of the heart. Well into the second half of the twentieth century, many doctors prescribed tablets made from digitalis leaf for congestive heart failure. Others who wanted a purer product used the alkaloid digoxin or a similar synthetic molecule.

A purer substance is not always most desirable. The side effects of other chemicals in the whole leaf indicated when the dose might be too strong for a particular patient. This provided a way of monitoring the amount needed. It might be similar to the difference between drinking red wine versus vodka. Before a person has too much wine, the aldehydes and other impurities can produce sleepiness or a headache. The person drinking vodka will consume much more alcohol and not get a severe hangover until the next day.

Various herbs have been used for centuries to treat illness. Witches, witch doctors, folk healers and ancient Chinese and East Indian traditionalists have helped many people. Healing might occur because of trust in the power of the healer as discussed in the chapter on the Mind-Body Connection. Sometimes nothing works. The wise physician in any culture treats the whole patient, learning about their diet, lifestyle and mental attitude and how these may affect one's medical condition. An herb, pill or surgical procedure might lessen symptoms but not get to their causes.

Andrew Weil M.D. combines modern Western medicine and ancient practices

I know first-hand that one of Dr. Weil's herbal suggestions works. In 1995 and 1996, I had episodes of moderately severe arthritis in one or both knees. I had to use crutches just to get around the house. I blamed the osteoarthritis in the right knee on being in a long-leg cast for months after a fall from a glacier years ago. Both knees had taken a beating from strenuous skiing one week a year in my forties and fifties. I was taking six to eight ibuprofen tablets a day. I could no longer ride a bicycle; using the brake while driving a car was often painful. Although my doctor said I could safely take up to 24 mg of ibuprofen a day, I didn't want to be dependent on pills.

When I heard Dr. Weil on a PBS program say ginger could help arthritis, I started using it. Here in California and in other parts of the country with an Asian population, most grocery stores sell ginger root in the produce section. I started using a piece of root about the size of my thumb sliced into tofu stir-fries, scrambled eggs or other dishes.

Within a few months I could ride my bicycle and only used a cane as an aid when going downhill on hikes. Now, I don't need the pain pills and rarely use a knee brace for active exercise. It seems that some ingredient in ginger acts on one of the eicosanoids or prostaglandins in a manner similar to ibuprofen, but results came slower. No matter that the active ingredient hasn't been isolated, ginger works for me.

Millions of people take supplements but don't tell their doctors about them

Supplements can affect the action of prescription drugs. The elderly father of a friend wondered why he didn't react normally to the heart medicine from his doctor that was supposed to regulate its rhythm. I found out he had been taking iron pills on his own to prevent "tired blood." When he stopped the iron, his heart was then able to contract normally. Most doctors don't take time to ask about the supplements a patient is taking. Patients are afraid the doctor won't approve so don't volunteer the information. According to an AARP survey in 2002, 52 percent of those over fifty took vitamins or other supplements every day. While trying to take control of their health, they can easily succumb to advertisements on the radio or on the Internet. In fact, Americans spend more than $18 billion a year on dietary supplements. Since these products don't need approval by the U.S. Food and Drug Administration, consumers don't know if they're effective or even safe.

If you're taking prescription drugs, tell your doctor about the supplements or over-the-counter medications you're taking on your own. There might be interactions that either depress the action of the drug or magnify it. One study showed that the herb St. Johns' wort, useful in mild cases of depression, made the drugs against AIDS or those used in chemotherapy less effective.

Take advice from newsletters on the Internet or in some health food stores that tout specific products with a grain of salt. One said the aspirin you take to prevent blood clots in your heart and brain might make you blind or cause a stroke. This disregards the dose. A baby aspirin, with less than one fifth of the salicylates of adult aspirin, safely prevents clots. Continued use of two or more regular aspirin a day can erode the tissues and cause bleeding in the gastro-intestinal tract or even in the brain. A little is good, more can be dangerous.

After hearing about secret herbal formulas on radio programs, I wouldn't send in $60 or more for a two-months supply of anything. The letters or contrived names of the substances mean nothing. The hucksters mainly tout testimonials and give poor or unscientific explanations of why their nostrum works. I'm always leery of combinations of active ingredients. You wouldn't know which might be causing side effects or even an allergy.

Taking evening primrose oil had unintended consequences

I read that gamma linolenic acid, an omega-3 fatty acid in evening primrose oil, has been used to relieve Raynaud's disease. In this condition, the vessels in the hands and feet clamp down in cold temperatures and make toes and fingers even colder. I have suffered with this since adolescence and hoped for a cure. I took this oil at night. I didn't notice any difference in my hand temperature when exposed to cold, but I slept more soundly and felt less stiff in the morning. However, about three weeks after starting the evening primrose oil, I noticed a dull ache in my left knee, relieved by 200 mg. ibuprofen. When I walked or went dancing I noticed a clicking of the cartilage of that knee -a new sensation. When I stopped the oil, the clicking and the pain were gone in a few days.

I read later that evening primrose oil can cause joint inflammation in some people. My response might relate to my specific body chemistry. A friend alternates two weeks of flax oil with two weeks of evening primrose oil. Flax oil has _alpha_ linolenic acid that controls eicosanoids that protect against auto-immune diseases such as rheumatoid arthritis. Evening primrose oil has the slightly different _gamma_ linolenic acid. Just because both oils have omega-3 fatty acids and come from plants doesn't assure that either might not cause unusual side effects.

Natural combinations of chemicals in a particular plant might make them more effective

Natural foods often have substances that help the body get the best effect from the vitamin they accompany. The bioflavonoids in the white membranes of citrus fruits help you use vitamin C. Most doctors, chemists and nutritionists 50 years ago thought that "the purer a substance the better" in order to use a specific chemical for a certain effect. However, there is no moderator.

We now know that heroin or morphine are much more addicting than the impure spirits of laudanum that old pharmacists extracted from poppies. Similarly, sniffing cocaine is more dangerous than chewing coca leaves, as the Peruvians have been doing for centuries. Purer might not be better. Some doctors still prescribe digitalis leaf for congestive heart failure instead of the pure active ingredient. Natural thyroid hormone from animal glands is often prescribed for thyroid deficiency and preferred by some patients to a synthetic chemical. The main advantage of synthetics is that they have been standardized as to dose and purity—important if you need an individualized dose.

Take the smallest amount of a supplement that gives the effect you want

In general, more is not better. Many books of herbal remedies have long lists of treatments for each ailment. It's like one of your children giving excuses. If there are too many of them, maybe none is very effective. Those that show pictures of the actual plants must want to avoid lawsuits, because they tell about severe symptoms or deaths from overdoses. It makes you wary of trying any of them. Modify someone else's recommendation as to how much of a substance to take. You are an individual and will have to find what is right for your body.

Nutritional Pharmacology edited by Gene Spiller gives examples of people who took too high doses of vitamins and minerals and suffered unintended side effects. *American Medicinal Plants* by Charles Millspaugh is along the same line. The book has good illustrations and tells of past uses of the herbs. Many write-ups end with a case of someone who used too much and got very sick or died.

Starting in 1790 and well into the nineteenth century, Dr. Samuel Hahnemann pursued the idea of giving tiny doses of the drugs of his era that were just enough to mimic certain disease symptoms, fever for example. He figured they would activate the body to mobilize its own defenses. He published a book in 1810 and the branch of medicine called "homeopathy" was born. His small homeopathic doses were much less dangerous than giving too much of a powerful medicine. They were also better than the purging or blood-letting that was popular with other doctors at that time. Even if it only gives a placebo response, a little is better than too much of anything. Students at Hahnemann Medical School in Philadelphia receive conventional medical training now but do learn about homeopathy.

I recommend the well-organized, encyclopedic book *Nutraceuticals*. Paragraph headings for each supplement include: Common Uses, How it Works, Evidence of Efficacy, Sources, Forms and Usual Dosages, Potential Problems and What to Look For. Historical notes accompany some of the write-ups. A long section in the book lists common disorders from acne to ulcers with possible remedies. This book makes walking into a health food store with its hundreds of possible health products less daunting.

Note that manufactured pills and capsules have standard doses, while the loose leaf or powdered root to be used as a tea might have variable concentrations of the active ingredients. Most vitamin C is made in a chemical laboratory. I don't believe that vitamin C extracted from rose hips and subjected to possible heat and pressure to make an expensive pill is superior to chemically produced ascorbic acid. The main difference between naturally extracted and chemically produced substances is that in the chemical process, you get both right-handed and left-handed forms of the molecule. If the body can use only one form, the rest would be excreted. The molecule from plants would have only the correct configuration so the body might use it all. Any excess would still go to the bladder unused. As mentioned before, it's best to get vitamins in natural foods.

Should the supplement industry be regulated?

In 1994, Congress tried to get the FDA to regulate supplements just as it does prescription drugs. This legislation never passed, as millions of Americans wrote to Congress and said they wanted to decide themselves what vitamins or other substances to take for their own health. A more palatable Dietary

Supplement Health and Education Act passed through Congress. It stated that dietary supplements were not to be treated as though they were unapproved drugs. Senators Tom Harkin of Iowa and Orrin Hatch of Utah asked for funding for research on alternative remedies.

Controlled studies so far show only that acupuncture prevents nausea and helps in dental pain. Meanwhile, the supplement industry has grown from $10 billion a year to $18 billion per year as American consumers continually hope for a magic pill. Both supplement makers and drug companies now sell more products. Many of these just treat symptoms.

More recently, after publicity about an athlete who died on a hot day after taking the herbal stimulant Ephedra, senators Richard Durbin of Illinois and Charles Schumer of New York introduced a bill requiring manufacturers of supplements to report adverse effects to the FDA. Deaths from supplements are tiny compared to 90,000 to 160,000 deaths per year from prescription and over-the-counter drugs, as reported by Donald Dyall in the summer, 2003 issue of *Health Freedom News*.

You must inform yourself about the side effects of over-the-counter pills or supplements

Tom was lucky to have survived the internal bleeding caused by his daily use of adult aspirin and the ibuprofen that relieved his chronic back pain. He apparently ignored warnings on the bottles that either could cause gastrointestinal bleeding. He treated his own chronic back pain and was able to do vigorous exercise in his late seventies. On a recent physical, his doctor found that his blood had very low hemoglobin. He saw two damaged discs in Tom's spine on x-ray. Tom had to have a spinal fusion operation that might mean the end of recreational sports, but he is alive. He should have used baby aspirin for his heart to prevent blood clots and a minimum of other pills. The many supplements he took over the years had not prevented the damage from his pain-killers.

One reason I wrote this book is to spread the word about the healing effects of ginger that got me away from taking ibuprofen for arthritis. By one estimate, 15,000 deaths a year from bleeding are caused by aspirin, ibuprofen or other NSAIDs (non-steroidal anti-inflammatory drugs), including Naproxen and Celebrex according to the AARP Bulletin.

Price and complexity are not necessarily a guide to the effectiveness of a treatment. Frontline, a 2003 PBS program, featured an alternative healer who has helped patients who hadn't been healed by conventional medicine or treatments. The fact that an initial consultation costs $2,800 and the regimen requires the patient to take 150 different pills a day along with six coffee enemas makes me wonder: Is the healer producing a strong placebo effect because of the complexity and cost and of his treatment? Is it like women's cosmetics? Expensive ones from a department store are used more faithfully than those from a drug store.

In a later chapter on the mind-body connection, I tell about a man known as the goat doctor of the Sierra. He healed hundreds of thousands of people who had also given up on the medical profession. However, he lived simply, used natural methods and didn't ask for an inflated fee.

You have to take charge of your own health

Read all you can and consult a reliable book such as *Nutraceuticals.* When buying a supplement in the health food store, try to stay with one herb and not a mixture. If something goes wrong, you want to know what caused the problem. You might be allergic to one of the ingredients. You might have unusual side effects from another. Look into nutraceuticals and other supplements but buy them and try them with care.

It's usually best to start slowly with less than what the bottle says is a normal daily dose. You might have to take them for months to get healthier skin or hair or to have more energy. Keep a diary of what you're taking and observations on relief of symptoms and possible side effects. Be aware that many herbs take a few weeks to show results. A supplement that works too quickly might have a stimulant like ephedra that can be dangerous. If you notice no difference after using one herb, then try another. You must be your own guinea pig. In summary, try one product at a time and give it several weeks to work

Meanwhile, concentrate on exercise and a natural diet to give your body a chance to heal itself. You must build your health on a solid foundation, then use just enough supplements to help your body keep it well. Some authors suggest taking 20 or 30 types of supplements a day. That's almost as bad as taking 10 or more prescription pills like many elderly people do now. Your own body's cells can and do make many of the important chemicals contained in supplements. You can get their miraculous effects as long as you're eating a balanced natural diet and getting enough exercise.

Aim for the Golden Mean.

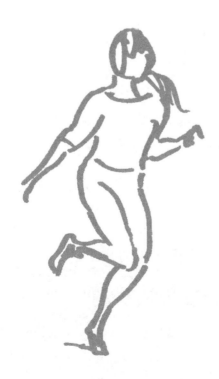

What You Can Do.

- Take a minimal dose multivitamin, multimineral pill daily or every other day.

- Consider taking a higher dose of these at night after extreme exertion, since your body repairs itself when you're asleep.

- Take more antioxidants if you're in a polluted environment.

- Try special supplements for individual problems, after first eating a good healthy diet of natural foods, especially green vegetables and brightly colored vegetables and fruits.

- Use egg yolks, wheat germ, brewers' yeast, flax oil and black molasses for extra nutrition.

- Be sure you're getting enough magnesium with your added calcium every day.

- If you're on hormones, take the smallest dose that gives the desired result.

- Try vitamins or amino acids instead of expensive or dangerous drugs.

- Use vitamins B-6, B-12 and folic acid to lower homocysteine to prevent heart attacks.

- See if specific amino acids can correct deficiencies in brain chemicals and combat other problems as shown in the chapter on Allergies and Addictions.

- Take some extra vitamins, minerals and antioxidants but remember the Golden Mean and don't use excessive amounts.

Exercise

*You might want to lose weight, improve muscle
tone or look better.*

We have muscles for a reason. In the past, a young, firm, lithe or muscular body helped attract a mate. Since we're living beyond our reproductive years, it is a matter of personal pride to be fit and trim.

15-1 Reasons to exercise

You need exercise for general health

Inactivity is much worse than too much exercise. However, there is more to life than having a perfect body. It seems as bad to build your life around your jogging schedule as to build it around an excessive work schedule. Strive for balance in your life. The ancient Greeks said you need both a sound body and a sound mind. Exercise can improve both body and brain.

Surplus food began with agriculture along the Nile about 7,000 years ago. The Drs. Eades book *Protein Power* disputes the idea that everyone was lean like those in ancient Egyptian paintings. Some mummies had loose skin, larger in area than the muscles under it because of fat under the skin. This was from eating grains, according to the Doctors Eades. Another explanation might be that these mummies were from a sedentary class that gained fat from inactivity.

A high-calorie diet combined with lack of exercise puts fat on any animal

Look at our feedlots where cattle or pigs are crowded together. The weight they gain is fat, not muscle, whether fed grain or high-protein soybeans.

An exercise specialist, Dr. Kenneth Epstein, says that our

children are being fattened like veal on a high-calorie diet with little exercise. According to Epstein, 13 percent of children 8 to 12 years old are already obese. Instead of playing outside after school, many sit inside in front of a television or a computer. Besides being inactive, they are eating snacks. Dr. Davis Stein estimates that children's television programs show more than 12 advertisements for fast food per hour versus three per hour in adult shows. He dramatizes the result of viewing 2,500 calories per hour by saying that every 60 seconds, a small child is asking a parent in a grocery store for some kind of junk food.

Back in the 1960s, there were few fat kids but many were flabby

The late President John F. Kennedy urged that fitness be a national goal. President George W. Bush, who runs and lifts weights, restored the President's Council on Physical Fitness early in his first term. He warns that deaths related to being sedentary and eating too much is approaching that of using tobacco.

Epstein urges parents to help their children not to form new fat cells. An old theory said that adults don't get new fat cells -those you got in childhood remain, begging to be filled. This convenient excuse might not be true. My two sisters were always thin as children and adolescents. Now they could each lose 30 pounds. I was a very chubby two-year-old. A spiteful neighbor told my mother I would grow up to be the fat lady in a circus. In later childhood, I was of medium weight. I got to 137 pounds in my thirties but when I stopped dieting, I dropped to around 120 and have maintained it for many years.

I'm a true believer in exercise, having overcome an early lack of coordination. I had failed all junior high school sports, but I started hiking and learned to swim in high school. In college, I learned to ski and to play all women's sports. I feel that gaining physical skills gave me confidence in other aspects of life. Swimming also relaxed my tired leg muscles after standing all day working in a laboratory. Hiking, swimming and other vigorous activities have helped me reduce the long-term stress of problems that once seemed overwhelming. They cleared my mind of negative thoughts. Strenuous movement also dissipated the dangers of short-term adrenaline stress hormones that our Paleolithic ancestors used for flight or to fight.

Active movement always works better to control weight than eating less fat or cutting total calories

On average, Americans gain a pound a year from their late twenties through their sixties. They don't eat more, just exercise less. Humans developed over many millennia, eating a varied diet accompanied by adequate exercise. According to the Center for Disease Control, 40 percent of Americans today are inactive. There may be fewer fat people in big cities than in small towns and suburbs. In older cities, you walk to a subway station and use the stairs rather than wait for an escalator. At the other end, you walk several blocks to your office. In a small town, you drive from home and park where you work. Suburban dwellers use automobiles even more. They buy fast food, visit banks and even mail packages while staying in their cars. Besides sitting all day, they sit around all evening. It's no wonder that over 60 percent are overweight.

Exercise charts show how many calories are used in various activities

To lose a pound of fat you would have to burn 3,500 extra calories. You can get discouraged trying to lose weight by doing rapid body movements. It makes sense to spend some time on exercises that build more muscle. Muscle burns calories even during sleep.

Start with walking. Your extra fat is like wearing a backpack. As your leg muscles become stronger, you can go farther and start to burn some of that body fat as you keep moving. Some authors say you should run or do similar aerobic exercise at least an hour a day, six days a week. That isn't necessary to achieve normal weight. Cut down on driving and walk as part of daily life. You can then add two to four hours of more vigorous exercise on weekends.

Exercise helps you avoid obesity and metabolic diseases, so it will

save you money

Medicare will be bankrupt if all the Baby Boomers don't start living healthier lifestyles. By 2010, there will be 40 million more people on Medicare. Costs already are more than $14 billion a year according to the Gray Panthers. Even now, the average person on Medicare spends another $1,964 yearly out of his own pocket, with sicker people paying $5,000 and often much more.

Forget the myths that say you can take specific pills to lose fat and build muscle without exercise

Body builders who take steroids and protein-derived chemicals such as carnitine use them in addition to exercise, not to replace it. Humans developed during hundreds of thousands of years by eating natural foods and doing vigorous exercise. No magic medicines or supplements can compare to these as a basis for a firm, healthy body.

Exercise can keep your bones strong so you won't fear falling

Many older people are so afraid of falling, they become less active and rarely go out. Trying to avoid something makes it more likely. Avoiding eggs causes your body to make more cholesterol. Cutting calories makes you eat more later. Becoming more sedentary makes it more likely that you'll suffer a broken bone if you fall.

Routine activities can put good stress on bones and muscles. Our grandmothers kneaded bread dough by hand. Now we have bread machines to get that home-baked flavor. Manufacturers urge us to get the lightest possible appliances. It might be better to get a heavy vacuum cleaner to carry from the closet to the carpeted areas. A hand-pushed reel mower to cut the lawn provides a lot more exercise and doesn't pollute the air like a gasoline mower.

Sports such as bowling, golf and tennis help the bones and muscles of the upper body. In San Diego, I knew women in their thirties, forties and fifties who strengthened their bones and muscles, especially in the upper body by taking up water-skiing or wind-surfing. Sports can be fun and make any chores seem easier as your muscles get stronger.

Sports, dancing, and exercises such as yoga and tai chi improve your balance so you don't fall in the first place. Your legs automatically react to prevent falling when you trip on something. Try standing on one foot while waiting in line at a store. The interplay of muscles helps your balance. Use more effort in all your daily activities to keep in shape and not be afraid of falling. A doctor can set a broken bone but you must make the conditions for the body to heal itself.

It is imperative for you to take care of yourself as the health care system changes. Corporations have bought community hospitals, then closed them if they didn't make enough money. Emergency rooms are more crowded as people lose health insurance. Even with Medicare, it's what you do yourself that determines how well you survive a fall. Prevention is better than cure.

Exercises should include aerobics, strength building and something for flexibility and balance

Any exercise is better than no exercise. The best is the one you do consistently, even if it doesn't have all needed components. It's even better if the exercise is fun and can be done with other people. It will broaden your social contacts and help your mental attitude. As your body gets healthier you will be able to increase the duration and type of exercise. It will produce a joy of living. As Dr. William Regelson says "Exercise is the closest thing we have to a fountain of youth."

15-2 Aerobic Exercise

Aerobic exercise is one way to increase physical activity

Vigorous aerobic exercise was popularized in the 1960s when Dr. Kenneth Cooper showed that bicyclists had healthier hearts than football players. Exercise is aerobic if the body takes in enough oxygen to completely burn cellular substances to form carbon dioxide and water. In anaerobic exercise, the muscles are used so strenuously they can't get enough oxygen so they just partially burn glucose. This is less efficient and the lactic acid produced can cause pain or muscular cramps. With rest, the lactic acid is oxygenated completely to carbon dioxide and water.

Jogging is considered the aerobic exercise anyone can do - good for the heart, lungs and blood vessels. Jogging isn't likely to cause chest pain if done slowly enough so you have enough breath to talk with your partner. Some doctors say you can just walk an equivalent distance. This might be almost as good for burning calories but it wouldn't put optimum stress on your heart.

Depending on your age, you should raise your heart rate up to 65 percent to 85 percent of its maximum in order to help your heart muscle get fit and stay fit. One rule of thumb for figuring the absolute maximum is to subtract your age from 220. A 30-year old with a maximum of 190 could strive for 85 percent of this or 162 beats per minute. A 70-year-old wouldn't want to exceed 80 percent of 150, or 120 beats per minute, after getting in shape. If sedentary, he could start with the 65 percent goal of 98 beats per minute.

An average heart rate at rest is between 70 and 80. A fit person with a well-developed muscular heart can have a resting rate under 50. One measure of cardiovascular fitness is how quickly your heart gets back to its resting rate when you stop the exercise. This can happen in less than a minute. For an accurate reading of your rate with exercise, take your pulse as soon as you stop and for only 10 seconds. Multiply this by 6 to get beats per minute. Even better: count beats per six seconds times 10. Decide for yourself if it's quicker to feel an artery in your wrist or at your neck just to the side of your windpipe.

A *sprint is anaerobic*

The runner goes so fast that he can't get enough oxygen to his muscles until the sprint is over. When I taught physiology, I explained the difference between two types of muscle fibers. Those that help in anaerobic exercise contain a lot of glycogen like the white meat in a chicken. The large breast muscles attached to the wings enable the chicken to quickly fly over a fence or up in a tree out of the reach of a predator. The red muscles in a chicken's legs allow it to walk or run around all day on the ground.

A wild duck, on the other hand, has red fibers in all its muscles. The red indicates a good blood supply so the duck can continue to metabolize body fat and get it to the muscles used in flying. The whole flight is aerobic, with adequate oxygen to continue for hours at a time. With a better blood supply, individual cells of exercising muscles are stimulated to make more mitochondria. These are the tiny furnaces inside cells that combine the break-down products of food with oxygen to produce energy. No pill or supplement can build them. A person has to move his muscles to stimulate more mitochondria that use more oxygen. A sprint won't help since it just increases the enzymes in muscle cells that partially burn glucose.

A way to compare exercises is to quantify the amount of oxygen used per minute

We can use METs (metabolic equivalents). Researchers hook subjects to an air tank and measure the amount of oxygen used while doing various activities. One MET is the volume of oxygen burned per minute when someone is sitting quietly. (A 155-pound young male uses about two-and-a-half quarts of oxygen. This would be different in others.) Moderate walking uses 3.5 MET while brisk walking is 4.5 MET. Jogging is between 6 and 10 MET, with running at 13 MET. Just as with heart rates, the maximum oxygen used varies with a person's age, sex and fitness level.

Most runners think all their energy is from muscle and liver glycogen that becomes glucose

This isn't good for a long run. A woman might have less than 1,400 calories and a man only 1,800 calories worth of glycogen to draw from. To get his glycogen stores as full as possible, a runner eats lots of carbohydrates the night before and more carbohydrates before a race, a process called carbo-loading. During a run, he drinks a source of more carbohydrates. If that isn't possible, something happens. He might get a cramp from lactic acid in his muscles, or feels weak and tired. He either gives up or realizes he's getting a second wind. His new energy comes from his body fat.

Some physiologists say to forget carbohydrate-loading. Pace yourself so you're burning a mixture of glycogen and fat from your body from the beginning. Both nutrients will be oxidized completely to carbon dioxide and water and you can last for hours. The Tarahumara Indians of the Sierra Madre in Mexico have been doing so for centuries. Runners should not try to decrease their body fat to 5 percent or less. They won't have the reserves for a long run that the person with more fat has. Since two to three pounds of special fat is never burned by the body, a 180-pound-man with 5 percent fat has six pounds of fat available for energy. The runner with 10 percent fat has 15 pounds of fat available to burn. Complete body stores of glycogen at 4 calories a gram yield 1,400-1,800 calories of energy. Fifteen pounds (6,800 grams) of fat at 9 calories per gram produce 61,000 calories of energy for a long distance run. Your muscles do not require carbohydrates during exercise. In fact, if your muscles have plenty of blood vessels like the wild duck, you burn body fat long after reserves of glycogen are gone.

Fat is the preferred fuel for the heart and other muscle cells

It's a myth that you get energy for movement only by the burning of carbohydrate. Carbohydrates are good for quick energy as in a sprint, but burning fat can sustain the body over the long haul. If you haven't eaten fat, your stores of body fat are used for energy. Two-carbon fragments break off from long chains of fatty acids. These are burned as active-acetate in the tiny mitochondria inside the cells. A balanced higher calorie diet metabolizes body fat during exercise. Fit muscles also burn fat at rest. Eat fat the day before a strenuous run and afterward to replace your body fat. Proteins, however, are not an efficient source of energy. First their amino groups must be removed to be excreted as urea. Then the resultant molecules are metabolized like carbohydrates to carbon dioxide and water.

You need a balance of fat, protein and carbohydrate

Just before strenuous exercise choose carbohydrates since they require less digestion than proteins and fat. After exercise you need protein and fat to repair your muscles. Runners who think a healthy diet has 70 to 80 per cent carbohydrates, and only 10 to 15 percent each of fat and protein have been misled. They can be thin but not healthy if they don't get enough essential fats to make cell membranes and sex hormones. Even saturated fats in the diet can be burned for energy to spare body fat. Runners need enough proteins to build the substances in their immune systems. It's no wonder that runners often get more colds and women can get thin, brittle bones and even quit menstruating.

If you eat a balanced diet you won't be dependent on extra vitamins and special supplements along with six meals a day. Runners can aim for the Golden Mean of 20-30 percent each of protein and fat and only 40-60 percent carbohydrate. Moderate exercisers would need less carbohydrate.

A sedentary person can't expect good health no matter what they eat or don't eat

Limiting carbohydrates might decrease body fat but does little to combat aging or prevent many metabolic maladies. Any exercise is better than none. Walking is something anyone can do. Many books say to walk 30 minutes a day, five times a week. This needn't be in one session. It could include walking to public transportation instead of driving. You can walk up stairs instead of taking the elevator. When you drive to go shopping, park so you walk several hundred feet across the parking lot.

A simple method for getting more exercise is to count all the steps you take during the course of your day. The goal of 10,000 steps a day can be measured by wearing a pedometer strapped to a belt or in a pocket. A group in Denver started with a goal of 2,000 steps a day, less than a mile, and kept increasing. Getting in extra steps can also help make some chores seem less onerous.

You would get up to switch television channels instead of using a remote control. You would gladly take walks with your children or your dog. You can modify your walking in the house by using different muscles. Hold your shoulders back in an exaggerated posture to prevent the rounded back that often comes with age. Walk on tip-toe to strengthen your feet and ankles.

Exercise can compensate for a diet called "unhealthy" by anti-fat purists

An article by David Bassett in the January 2004 issue of *Medicine & Science in Sports and Exercise* analyzed the diet and exercise of an Amish community in Canada, where just 4 percent were obese and only 26 percent even overweight. Contrast this with two-thirds of those in the U.S. in these categories. The Amish eat like our grandparents - meat, potatoes, eggs and dessert plus seasonal vegetables. Without modern conveniences, everyone walked and farmed without motorized equipment. According to pedometers, the men averaged 18,425 steps a day and women averaged 14,196 steps.

A long-term cardiac fitness study using a treadmill was reported by Steven Blair in a 1995 article in the Journal of the American Medical Association. He says that fit men had a death rate of 39.6 per 10,000 man-years, while the unfit rate was 122 deaths. The unfit, who then went on an exercise program, cut the death rate of that group to 67.7. Each minute more in maximum treadmill time produced a 7.9 percent decrease in mortality. Exercise is much more important than diet or total cholesterol levels since it raises the "good" HDL cholesterol.

You can't expect exercise to correct all conditions

Runner Jim Fixx probably overdid his running in the attempt to increase the coronary blood supply to his heart. He may not have known that other factors such as too much homocysteine or the presence of *Chlamidiae pneumonia* bacteria can cause fatty deposits in blood vessels. Nicotine, too-high insulin or high blood pressure can also cause injuries to the blood vessel walls that are then patched with cholesterol and fat. You want to get healthy, not become a dead exercise fanatic.

Jogging can be harmful if overdone

As mentioned already, some women runners lose too much body fat thus decreasing their estrogen and making their bones like those of a sedentary crone. Too much running can also depress the immune system and make a person prey to viruses and bacteria. Covert Bailey in *Fit or Fat* says the runners with most injuries are those who run more than 35 miles a week. More is not better. You might be healthier by running only every other day. Don't run at all if you think you might be coming down with a cold.

Walking and jogging are the simplest aerobic exercises

For some people, walking their dog gets them out once or twice a day whatever the weather. Catherine, who has been on crutches from a chronic condition, says she gets more exercise because of her small trained "service dog." The dog makes sure she gets up in the morning, always does some walking and takes her medication. In fact, she now needs fewer pain pills because of the dog.

In order to help your cardio-vascular system, any aerobic exercise has to make your heart beat faster than when you're sedentary. As a person becomes more fit, his resting pulse is slower as his heart beats more strongly and efficiently. However, walking or jogging doesn't exercise all the leg muscles, much less the upper body. Hiking or bicycling uphill uses the thigh muscles as well as the calf muscles. The more any muscle is used the better it can burn both carbohydrates and fats.

When I can't go on a four- to six-hour Sierra Club hike, I go up and down some steep trails that branch off from a local equestrian path. College runners can race up the 15 to 30 degree slopes, but I get my pulse rate high enough by hiking. Since I'm wearing my heaviest boots (five pounds), I feel I'm getting a more complete workout than if I jogged on the nearly flat bicycle trail wearing light-weight shoes.

The best exercise is the one you enjoy and keep doing. In Sacramento, a senior program called "Dance for Life" caters to those over 60. It includes two afternoon sessions of ballroom dancing with a half-hour dance lesson. There are several mixers and the opportunity to socialize. Even though the dancing is not very strenuous, it's as good as or better than walking. One couple in their eighties can outdo younger participants with their artistic and lively variations to basics such as the fox-trot and waltz, as well as many Latin American dances.

Besides helping your muscles, heart, coordination and balance, exercise can be good for your brain

Exercise causes the growth of more memory cells, according to Dr. Victoroff in *Saving Your Brain*. He says that 30 minutes of moderate exercise five times a week or 20 minutes of vigorous exercise three times a week is optimum to prevent problems of an aging brain. Victoroff says that aerobic exercise is better than strength training to increase "fluid intelligence," the ability to adapt and learn from new experiences. Exercise not only helps you keep your brain power as you get older, but helps form new nerve cells in the parts of the brain that help co-ordination and memory.

15-3 Weight Training

You can increase the size of your muscles by doing some form of weight training

Body-building with weights enlarges muscles by increasing the size of individual fibers. This is limited by your natural body hormones. Muscle tissue uses calories whether a person is exercising, sitting or asleep. A pound of muscle needs 10 times more calories at rest than does a pound of fat. So if you have a limited amount of time for exercise, it makes more sense to spend some time building more muscle instead of just trying to use up more calories by walking or running. A pound of fat contains 3,500 calories. If jogging uses 500 calories per hour, it would take seven hours to lose that pound of fat.

There are gyms all over the country where men and an increasing number of women use either free weights or those attached to machines to build muscle. However, machines aren't a necessity. More than 70 years ago, Charles Atlas transformed himself from a skinny weakling to a well-muscled man. He called his system Dynamic Tension, in which opposing muscle groups work against each other or against gravity to build muscle.

Many men use machines in a gym and also consume protein powders and other substances, including anabolic steroids. These supplement their natural muscle-building testosterone. They do get bulky muscles, but not necessarily more useful muscles. They won't be pushed around by strangers but the extra hormones might make them too aggressive. I once cut in front of a car driven out of the parking lot of a gym. The hulking man got out of his car at the traffic light and said he would have hit me in the face if I weren't an old lady. Steroid overuse can also harm a man's liver and kidneys. Women who try for large muscles by using steroids look grotesque to me.

Three types of muscle activities are involved in weight training

A contracted muscle gets shorter. This is called concentric. It is isometric when the muscle stays the same length but exerts force in resisting a stress. It is eccentric when the muscle lengthens slowly after a contraction but resists the force of gravity. The best one to build muscle is the sustained release eccentric action. In doing push-ups, slowly let yourself down for maximum benefit. You also notice the eccentric action when going down a long flight of stairs. You feel the descent more in your thigh muscles even though walking upstairs, a concentric activity, requires more energy.

Downhill skiing can use all three actions. Water-skiing requires mainly isometric action in your forearm muscles as you strain to hold the tow-rope. All three types of muscle action in legs, abdomen and back are used to get up out of the water on a single ski at the beginning of a run. Carrying a heavy suitcase would be an isometric activity. If your arm is bent, you use your biceps muscles, but the triceps are used with a straight arm. Muscles used in isometric activities are often stronger and tougher than those used in concentric or eccentric actions.

Most women can benefit from weight training

Dr. Miriam Nelson in her book *Strong Women Stay Young* dispels the idea that women build huge muscles just by using weights. Their low level of natural adrenal testosterone doesn't promote this. However, women at any age can build strong useful muscles. Knowing that several studies showed that older men could build muscle, Nelson recruited a group of 40 post-menopausal women to see if they could be helped as well. All were healthy but sedentary, and none were on replacement hormones. The results were astounding. The women doing strength training gained bone density while the control group continued losing bone calcium. The women on strength training were energized. Their balance improved 14 percent, while the controls declined 8.5 percent. Best was the fact that all in the exercise group lost inches and needed smaller dress sizes as their bodies were toned and tightened and muscle replaced fat. A 76-year-old even lost 29 pounds of fat. Nelson thinks that the increased bone density and improved balance that goes along with stronger muscles will keep her group from being among the 30 percent of people over 70 who break their hips and need extensive hospitalization.

Using exercise machines

Nelson used exercise machines in her study because they produced numerical values. She says that anyone can get similar results using dumbbells and ankle weights. Even exercises without weights, where a woman uses her muscles against the force of gravity, such as doing push-ups, can be useful. Magazine articles suggest using soup cans as weights but they aren't heavy enough. Muscles must work to 80 percent of their maximum over two sets of eight repetitions to get stronger. As soon as an exercise seems easy at a certain weight, the person must go to heavier weights.

In Nelson's program, women do eight exercises for 40 minutes twice a week using weights. The muscle is contracted slowly over three seconds, held two seconds then slowly extended over another three seconds. Sessions could be broken into 20-minute segments as long as muscles have two days to recuperate. It isn't good to wait until the weekend and then lift weights both days.

The book has excellent drawings, often of an older, slightly plump woman. Get the book for an explanation of the types of weights, repetitions and progression to heavier weights. Her exercises include lifting alternate straight legs while sitting to strengthen the muscles at the front of the thigh. In other exercises, you stand holding the back of a chair, while lifting the ankle-weighted legs to the side or straight back. These help strengthen hip and buttock muscles and those on the back of the thigh. Strengthen arm and shoulder muscles by using dumbbells while seated.

I met a woman, probably in her thirties, who looked trim and slender. She wasn't eating any of the fabulous food at a *Mardi Gras* party because she said she was competing that weekend in a body-building contest. I observed that with her high proportion of muscle, she could probably eat three times as much as the average woman. She replied that she can, but to keep the definition of muscle groups favored by the judges, she can't eat anything but low-calorie vegetables for the next few days. Most women who strengthen their muscles with resistance exercises don't get bulky muscles because they have only a low level of adrenal testosterone. Some of those who compete might be taking steroids so each muscle gets larger. If you're not on steroids, you can have strong useful muscles and be lithe and lean.

It is important to strengthen the triceps muscles on the back of the upper arm

These muscles are often flabby even on younger women. My triceps muscles got stronger when I used crutches for seven months as an isometric activity resisting gravity. Now a good triceps exercise for me is a modified push-up while standing behind my couch. I lean my straight body forward until my head touches the back of the couch between my hands. I straighten my arms in five counts, hold the straight body position five counts, then lower my body for 10 counts until my head is at the level of my hands. Fast push-ups are much easier than those where you slowly let yourself down. Younger people can do the typical straight body push-ups off the floor. You could also try modified push-ups where you kneel on the ground.

Deepak Chopra and David Simon, in *Grow Younger, Live Longer,* describe seven basic strength-building exercises. First, sit while holding the dumbbells of appropriate weight. Curls contract the biceps muscle as you lift a weight to shoulder level. Slowly straightening the arm holding the dumbbell is an eccentric activity. Other exercises with dumbbells strengthen the shoulder rotator muscles. Slow push-ups help all arm and shoulder muscles. Slow sit-ups or crunches strengthen the abdominal muscles. To strengthen back muscles, lie face down and try to raise the chest off the floor without pushing with the arms. Do slow partial knee bends for thigh muscles. Slowly rise onto the toes while holding a chair for balance to help ankle, foot and leg muscles.

Many weight-training programs talk about repetitions and sets of each exercise. Repetitions are the number of times a given weight is lifted without stopping and a set is the number of times you do reps (repetitions). "Max" means the maximum amount of weight you can lift at one time. "RM" means "repetitions max," the most repetitions you can do with that weight. Robert Quintana, Director of Performance Research at California State University, Sacramento says that if you can do 15 reps, the weight is too light. If you can do only five or six, it's too heavy. Adjust the weight so you can do 8 to 12 reps in good form. The first set would have more reps than the second or third.

In all weight training, you do the exercises slowly to make the muscles work hard. Then the individual fibers grow larger. This is different from calisthenics, where each movement is done rapidly many times to encourage the burning of energy. Both types of exercise are helpful in keeping your body in shape, but have different results.

Use your muscles as much as possible in daily activities. Manufacturers have done you a disservice over the years by making appliances ever lighter. Sometimes they don't even save time. With a lighter iron, you have to go over a piece of clothing more times to get out the wrinkles than with a heavier one. Plastic is lighter but seldom as durable as metal. I'm sorry now I traded my sturdy heavy Pfaff sewing machine for a lightweight Singer that doesn't work as well. At least the heavy manual typewriter I use for envelopes helps my muscles as I lift it onto the table. As much as possible, carry heavy groceries and use manual equipment in yard work or have an athletic hobby that requires some strain on the muscles. The more muscle tissue you have, the more calories you burn day and night. Join a gym or follow Miriam Nelson's program. Remember her motto: Strong women stay young.

15-4 Yoga for Health

Several types of yoga have developed over thousands of years in India and neighboring Asian countries. Yoga can be translated as "union"— the gaining of one-ness of body, mind, emotion and spirit. Most types of yoga practiced in Asian countries have a spiritual aspect and often include breathing and mindful meditation. Here in the West, physical aspects are practiced in what is called Hatha Yoga. Even this has several variations, but the whole body is used as well as explicit breathing exercises. Most Hatha Yoga is based on holding certain positions or *asanas*. Besides other benefits, yoga is creates flexibility.

In a light form of Hatha Yoga, practitioners do bends, twists and balances, holding the positions for a gentle stretch. The Iyengar style is stricter and emphasizes long holds. B. K. S. Iyengar, born in India in 1918, still practices yoga. His life is proof that it delays aging. His teaching methods integrate body and mind. He says that specific *asanas* can direct energy and blood flow into those parts of the body that are ailing and help the body to heal itself. This is better than taking pills that only relieve symptoms.

In yoga, the idea is to hold a position several seconds or even several minutes

This is different from calisthenics where you repeat a movement as rapidly as possible. Even without movement, muscles, tendons at the ends of muscles and the ligaments that hold the joints together are all subjected to a steady tension. In any yoga position, you should feel slight pain as you hold a position and know that the muscles, tendons and ligaments are being gently stretched. Don't bounce, as this might tear some muscle fibers. Be gentle and respect your body. Count your breaths as you hold a position and learn patience. Sometimes it takes months to achieve the correct position.

Yoga is mostly isometric to keep muscles toned and taut. It also aids in flexibility and balance. *Asanas* done by standing on one foot stimulate an interaction of leg muscles to maintain balance. Depending on how much the body must resist gravity to hold a position, yoga can help prevent osteoporosis. It's most effective when done in addition to strength training and aerobics.

Rodney Yee, instructor from Piedmont, California, says that yoga itself can be aerobic. After a quick 108 sun salutations, his heart rate will be as high as after a run or walking half an hour on a treadmill. He does a type of yoga called Ashtanga. It combines correct breathing with a flow of movements that creates inner body heat. Power yoga is an even more vigorous variant of this style.

Not everyone can be that dedicated. I would rather do a slow salute-to-the-sun even though it's supposed to be a continuous transition from one position to another. I feel I get a better stretch of back, groin and leg muscles and strengthening of arms and shoulders by holding each position first for 10 slow counts, then each for 20 or 30 seconds in the next set of repetitions. Even at this slow pace, if I'm in a cold room this exercise warms me enough so I must remove my sweatshirt.

Yoga twists, bends and extensions of the torso keep your spine flexible

It is important to alternate positions where the back is bent forward with ones where it is curved backward, allowing the two sets of opposing muscles to both get a workout. In the cobra position, you lie face down and while leaving the abdomen touching the ground slowly lift the torso by pushing down and trying to straighten the arms. In the beginning, you may be able to raise your chest only a few inches. As you practice week after week you can rise higher, lengthen your neck and feel like a cobra, strong and in control.

This pose is best followed by the resting-child position, where you kneel with a rounded back, body tucked into a ball, with hands near your feet. In a variation, your arms are stretched in front of you as in a salaam. Another variation is to keep your head down but grab your ankles and raise your buttocks. If your back muscles still feel strained, you can let the floor massage them by rocking back and forward like the end of a somersault.

For another back massage, tuck your bent knees toward your chest while lying on your back with arms stretched at shoulder level to either side. Keeping knees together, rotate them from one side to the other, touching the floor below your arms.

Other positions allow the hips and shoulders to go through a full range of movement. A very flexible person with little muscle strength can do an *asana* called the "full lotus." In this, the person sits on the floor and places each foot, sole up, on the opposite thigh. However, people with stronger muscles, usually men, can only sit in a simple cross-legged position. I could do a half lotus only with my right leg when it was very thin after losing muscle tone by being in a long-leg cast for months.

A person needs both strength and flexibility. Yoga teacher Rodney Yee is one person who does have well-developed muscles and still has the flexibility to do a full-lotus. This might be because as a young man he was a ballet dancer and he continues extensive stretching exercises.

Some positions can bring extra blood to a part of the body. A headstand or a shoulder stand where the legs extend vertically in the candle pose are said to benefit the thyroid gland in the neck as well as the pineal and pituitary glands in the head. The effect can be accentuated in the plow position where the hips are flexed so the straight legs extend over the head and touch the ground behind the head. Since my HMO doesn't want to give me thyroid hormones for a borderline hypothyroid condition, I am hoping that these shoulder stands will stimulate my own thyroid gland to be more active. As it is, my resting oral temperature is 96 to 97 degrees instead of the standard 98.6 F.

Different authors have different approaches to yoga for the elderly

Suza Francina's *The New Yoga for People Over Fifty* is the most amazing. Francina noticed that elderly people who practiced yoga didn't show common conditions like arthritis, osteoporosis, trouble with heart and lungs, confusion and other problems often considered a natural part of growing old. She developed a group of props, including bolsters, straps, back-bending benches, walls and wall ropes for her students and for convalescent patients. These props enabled persons as old as 70 and 80 to be safe and gain confidence as they learned yoga techniques. Francina's book has numerous photographs on the use of these aids. It's astounding to see old people doing handstands and back bends. The photos as well as the props encourage people who have been sedentary to gradually lose their stiffness. They can benefit from simple poses even if they don't aspire to the advanced ones. Francina says yoga also helps during menopause, "making hot flashes into cool breezes."

Peggy Cappy of Peterborough, New Hampshire realizes that yoga can be intimidating for persons who haven't exercised in years. In *Yoga for the Rest of Us,* she starts her elderly students with correct breathing and very simple movements while holding on to the back of a sturdy chair or even sitting. She says you have to start with deep abdominal breathing to oxygenate all body tissues.

Abdominal or diaphragmatic breathing is superior to chest expansion in taking a deep breath

Lowering the diaphragm, the big horizontal muscle between the chest and the abdominal organs, draws more air into the lungs. One instructor told us to pretend we were putting air into a balloon by puffing out our tummies to draw in the air while inhaling. Relax and the air goes out naturally. You have to wear loose clothing since a tight belt won't allow the full depression of the diaphragm. Back in the 1950s, women's fashions accentuated a tiny waistline. It wasn't as bad as the corsets of other eras but still harmed those who wore tight belts and took shallow chest breaths.

Diaphragmatic breathing normalizes the interactions of the sympathetic and para-sympathetic nerves that form a network in the abdominal area known as the solar plexus. This can increase the amount of DHEA hormones while decreasing cortisone-type stress hormones. It's no wonder that abdominal breathing during meditation decreases blood pressure.

I discovered years later that always trying to hold in my abdomen might have contributed to my Raynaud's disease. In this condition, much more common in women than men, the blood vessels in the hands clamp down, making them painfully cold. Finally, I learned bio-feedback, first attached to a machine at Kaiser Permanente and then at home holding two tiny thermometers. Abdominal breathing for five to 10 minutes warmed my hands by 10 to 20 degrees. In the laboratory, they went from 80 degrees to the middle 90s. Even in a cool room at home, my hand temperature has risen from the mid-60s or 70s to the low 90s. It's hard to maintain good new habits even when wearing loose clothing. The only time I practice is when I wake up during the night.

Relaxation and reduction of tension in body and mind is the prime component in one type of yoga

You just lie on your back on the floor with arms at the sides, palms up, and concentrate on abdominal breathing. If you feel a strain on your back, put a pillow under your feet or knees. Another variation is to lie with your torso flat but with your legs extending up a wall. Twenty minutes in one of these positions can reduce stress and lower blood pressure just as well as some forms of meditation where you sit with eyes closed reciting a mantra, a single work or sound. Even though this correct breathing wouldn't tone the muscles and stretch the ligaments as do forms of Hatha Yoga, it's better than a cocktail after a stressful day.

Look at books on yoga to see which might be within your present or future abilities. I started by watching the yoga classes of Richard Hittleman, then those of Lilias Folan on television. Some yoga programs are too early in the morning when many people feel too stiff. It's better to wait until your muscles have warmed up from routine activities. You can get better stretches without danger. If possible, sign up for a yoga class to learn the correct way to do various positions. Suza Francina uses the Iyengar method. Others concentrate on building strength. Most help you gain flexibility. If you start with yoga that teaches breath control and relaxation, you can later go to one where you hold a position.

Practice at home on non-class days. If your time is limited, do a few *asanas* in good form and hold them as long as possible rather than hurry through an entire routine every day. Do a slightly different set of exercises on alternate days and gain benefits like those of cross-training in sports. Try for 15 to 20 minutes of yoga most days with a longer session once a week. It doesn't need to be the same time every day. It's best for me before lunch or dinner. In the early morning, I feel too stiff. If I miss a day, I try for a longer session the next day. Hatha Yoga might be too energizing for some people just before bedtime. However, if you lie down and do abdominal breathing during the last 10 minutes, it can still be relaxing.

Yoga should be a total experience for body and spirit. Most of the time, don't try to do it while watching an unrelated television program. It's much more satisfying when done to music. Use your favorite soothing music and look at something from nature, maybe a bouquet or your backyard. As your body gets stronger and more flexible, you are preventing debilitating aging as well as looking more youthful and feeling younger. Best of all, yoga makes you feel more alive.

My Versions of a few Yoga Exercises

Salute to the Sun:

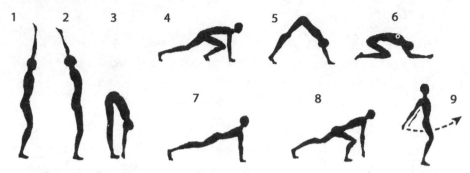

1. Stand tall, feet a little apart, Reach upward.
2. Bend slightly backward, buttocks pinched together to protect back, thumbs linked.
3. Bend down, keeping knees straight but not locked. Try to touch floor or grab ankles.
4. Extend one leg far backward. Sink down to stretch groin muscles. Forward knee is well bent.
5. Move other foot back, raise hips high. Start on balls of the feet; try to lower heels for tendon stretch.
6. Drop onto knees with hands in place. Tuck body into ball, head down. Get stretch of arms.
7. Move head and body forward so you're balancing on feet and hands with straight body. Raise head.
8. Bend one knee trying to move it forward close to the hands. Stand up with feet comfortably together.
9. Sweep arms forward then to side and back. Bend elbows and place palms together in front of chest.
10. Repeat sequence extending the other leg back. All the above positions should be held 10 seconds.
11. Repeat sequence again, holding each position 20 seconds.

Cobra:

1. Lie on your abdomen, feet somewhat apart, elbows bent, palms on ground near shoulders or ahead.
2. Press with arms trying to raise upper torso while keeping abdomen on the floor.

3. Hold position, then lower very slowly in 10 to 20 seconds.

4. Repeat, trying to raise higher and hold longer. Then again lower slowly to feel action of triceps.

Shoulder Stand

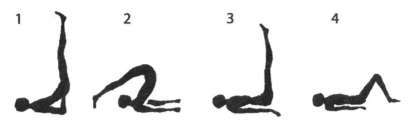

including Candle and Plow positions:

1. Lie on back, then roll up so hips are off the floor supported by hands. Feet extend upward. (Try to get as vertical as possible, though legs may angle toward the head.) Do ankle rotations in this position.

2. Extend one leg at a time over your head, trying to touch the floor.
   (If you're still too stiff, separate legs in a wide "V" and extend them over head, reaching toward floor.)

2a Return to upright shoulder stand, then try to put both legs together over your head to touch floor.

3. Return to upright and get more time in this position while massaging the front of the thighs.

4. Lower legs to a supine position (on back, face up). If your back is tired, roll back and forth like the end of a somersault.

Chest Opener

Benefits neck, back and shoulder muscles (useful to start session):

1. Stand with feet slightly apart. Clasp hands behind you. Straighten arms.

2. Try to raise hands high as possible as you're bending forward at the hips. Head up, chin leading.

3. Lower head to knees, with hands still clasped behind you.

4. Straighten up but try to raise hands & arms higher behind you.

5. Relax. Bend forward, knees slightly bent. Put hands on back of head.

6. Slowly straighten up while pushing on head with hands.

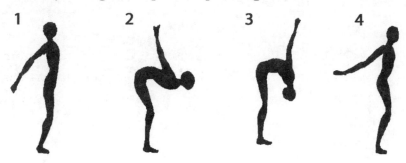

15-5 Other Types of Exercise

Anytime you move your body, you are exercising. When bigger muscles are moved, you get more exercise. During aerobic exercise, you oxygenate your heart, lungs and muscles. Weight training helps your muscles get larger and stronger. Yoga helps you keep your joints flexible, especially those in your back. It can also help your balance and relieve stress. Other types of exercise can also keep you healthy.

Gardening is the most popular hobby in the U.S. Gardening is the additional work you do in the yard besides cutting the grass with an automatic mower. It can provide light to heavy exercise, depending on what you do. It usually requires kneeling or stooping and might involve pushing a wheelbarrow with dirt or rocks or potted plants. It might include climbing a ladder to prune trees or bushes and to harvest fruit. It requires spading before planting.

Using various muscles in different body positions is equivalent to cross-training. It isn't as boring as using machines at a gym. You might not put maximum stress on all your muscles but you know you have used a lot of them. When working with plants, you feel like nature's partner. You see how your efforts help produce something beautiful or useful. This contrasts with many modern jobs, where your worth is measured by the number of items produced, the number of customers contacted or some intangible activity that earns dollars without satisfaction. We all originated as part of nature and our ancestors worked on the land. Get back to nature for better health.

Actively working with the earth can relieve stress as well as help your body. When I was the defendant in a frivolous lawsuit, I kept my sanity by digging up two-thirds of my large yard. I then planted fruit trees and replaced the sod with bark and vines. The trees produce fruit at different times of the year, uncontaminated by insecticides. Other vegetation helps absorb toxins from the ever-increasing smog in the Sacramento Valley. Yard work also helps keep my muscles in shape for windsurfing and other sports. Since it's difficult to lift my kayak to the roof of my new car, I shall use some of Nelson's strength training exercises. One of her patients was energetic at 89. Strong women stay young.

Harvey and Marilyn Diamond in *Fit For Life II* describe a gentle method of exercise. They say to jog, shuffle or bounce while standing on a rebounder (a mini-trampoline) while holding weights in your hands. Raising your hands in various positions should strengthen arm, shoulder, back and chest muscles. The sandbag weights couldn't be more than a couple of pounds, not enough to build much muscle. The best aspect of the rebounder is to gain or maintain a sense of balance.

Balance usually declines with age

One test I tried at a health fair involved walking on a squishy mat. It seems easy with eyes open, but difficult when they are closed. You can test your balance by standing on one foot with eyes closed and raise the other foot about four inches. Be careful and do it near a wall you can reach out and touch if you start to wobble. It's amazing how much we depend on our eyes for balance. A yoga exercise where you stand on one foot and bend the knee of the other leg and rest that foot on the inner thigh of the standing leg helps balance. Opposing sets of the muscles of the standing leg are activated to prevent swaying.

Any movement of the body is better than none as you get older. It can start slowly and doesn't have to be vigorous. One study of frail elderly people in a nursing home had them start with simple exercises where they tried to stretch and rotate their limbs while sitting. As they gained flexibility, they were able to stand and then began using weights. It would be an unusual nursing home where there is enough staff to help the elderly stand to exercise, much less use weights. Maybe teenage volunteers could be trained to help patients do simple movements while sitting, then to stand up and do gentle sustained movements like those practiced by old people in the parks in China.

At dawn in a park in the city of Luoyang, China, I had the chance to see and join a variety of exercise groups moving to the sounds of different taped music. Younger people did fast repetitive movements to Western music, while their elders were performing *tai chi*, an ancient sustained type of exercise. They went through a series of slow graceful movements that look inconsequential if not done right. By maintaining muscle tension, the people were doing isometric exercises. They kept their muscles toned and put their joints through a full range of movement.

If you have been sedentary for years, start with moderate walking and lifting small loads

It's good to have a standard routine, such as walking the dog, but you need a variety of body movements with different degrees of effort some of the time. Your bones and muscles are most strengthened by vigorous movements. Weekend exercisers are helping their bodies as long as they don't injure themselves by doing too much both days.

A muscle improves by any activity that gives it a degree of strain, as long as it has time to heal the inevitable micro-tears in the fibers. After a day of vigorous activity, you should take a multivitamin, multimineral tablet at bedtime. The body repairs itself when you're asleep. Take antioxidants before a major exercise session in polluted air.

Calisthenics have produced fitness in athletes and young recruits. Doing a vigorous exercise as fast as possible helps bring more blood to the muscles, as well as decreasing reaction time for a specific movement. This is important on both the athletic field and the battlefield. It can be boring for older adults. Active exercise done to music has been popular with women for years, whether called Jazzercise, Dance Aerobics or something else.

Even though it might not do much for strength or flexibility, it provides a good aerobic workout.

Pilates is a newly popularized form of exercise that builds strength, concentrating on the abdomen

This form of exercise was started by Joseph Pilates in England to help rehabilitate patients after World War I using special equipment. Later, he developed exercises that are done on the floor or while standing. The idea is to first strengthen the core muscles in the abdomen so you can stand tall and prevent a fat belly. Some instructors include using a large ball that you lie on to get interaction of muscles as you try to balance.

Denise Austin in *Pilates for Every Body* shows 18 to 36 slow exercises for the beginner to the advanced student. These tone and tighten muscles in all parts of the body as you work against gravity. Exercisers spend most time on the lengthening of the muscle after an original contraction. Austin ends with her selected yoga positions in a cool-down phase. Some Pilates instructors introduce fast movements that can be aerobic. One friend says that when he can't go jogging outdoors, he does Pilates exercises indoors.

Cliff Sheats in *Lean Bodies Total Fitness* uses both aerobics and strength training. He says you should increase the intensity of both to get your body tuned up to burn more body fat and build more muscle. In an eight-week "Lean Bodies" program, the first week has three 20-minute aerobic sessions and two sessions of weight training with light weights each day. By the eighth week, there are three daily 45-minute sessions of intense jogging or running and two sessions of using the heaviest weights you can handle in good form, doing 15 repetitions for each muscle group.

Women use lighter weights than men, but both are building muscle and losing fat. The accompanying diet is unusual. Women add 100 extra daily calories each week, going from a base of 1,500 calories to 2,200 calories per day. Men start at 2,000 calories and increase 200 calories a day each week to 3,400 calories per day.

People who have the time, the access to weight equipment and scrupulously follow the six meals a day diet can get astounding results, but then what? Must you continue the regimen forever? Would you have friends other than those on the jogging path or the gym? Will you be using those well-toned muscles for useful work and enjoyable athletic activities or are they just to look at?

A friend in his middle eighties has kept his good muscles for years without such a program. He worked for years as a brick layer and often had a second job, since he needs only four hours sleep a night. He has a girlfriend half his age and his main athletic activity is ping-pong. He gave me his videotape showing the 20 minutes of exercises he does daily. Since the moderate stretches and calisthenics are not too strenuous, his routine would be a good start for anyone. He doesn't trust doctors and won't let them do the special blood tests that might show why he isn't aging like his peers. At least he uses his muscles to help other seniors, like wielding a heavy chain saw to help trim branches off a tree. The rest of us don't have his unusual constitution. We have to eat a healthy diet and do a variety of exercises to get strong muscles and a flexible body.

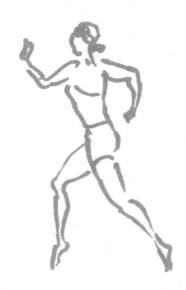

What You Can Do

- Start walking. Don't drive if you can walk. Use the stairs. Buy a pedometer to try for 10,000 steps a day. Take a walk instead of a snack.

- If you have been sedentary, keep a daily record of the minutes or hours you spend in any movement. Try to increase it every week. Vary your exercise program.

- Keep your heart and lungs in shape with aerobic exercise that gets your heart beating faster. Jogging, walking or bicycling uphill combines aerobic exercise with some strength building.

- Build muscle strength by exercising against resistance once or twice a week, using machines, dumb bells and ankle weights, slow calisthenics, or heavy lifting in work or play. Try for all three actions: concentric, isometric and eccentric. Do most yard work without machines.

- Keep your joints flexible with slow sustained exercises such as yoga or tai chi. Put each joint through its full range of motion every day.

- Do something that helps your balance such as standing on one foot while waiting in line. Do yoga or try tai chi exercises. Go dancing, play tennis or other sports.

- Have fun. Exercise with other people whether dancing, playing sports, hiking, doing exercises or in other active recreational activities.

- Feel the joy of being alive without debilitating aging as you exercise the rest of your life.

- Don't let compulsive exercise be the most important part of your time on earth. Do enough but not too much. Remember the Golden Mean.

Alternative Therapy & The Mind-Body Connection

*Exercise, diet and supplements can all affect
a person's body chemistry and sometimes,
his brain chemistry. Even this is a general
statistical average. We are individuals and
might react differently to the same chemicals.*

As advised earlier, use the smallest amount of a supplement that relieves your symptoms. As you feel healthy, you might be able to stop using it. Besides moderate to vigorous exercise and a natural balanced diet, you need to control stress and negative thinking. You can use your brain to help your body. In fact, I have friends who have each survived two different types of cancer within 10 years. Both have a positive outlook and something worth living for.

Alternative therapies can affect both body and brain

Dr. Kenneth R. Pelletier in *The Best Alternative Medicine* discusses complementary and alternative medicine (CAM) as an adjunct to conventional medicine. He says it is hard to analyze these unconventional treatments. The healers treat their patients as individuals who can't be matched with someone else. They don't think it's ethical to give any of them a placebo. The closest they come to following the scientific method is to give alternate patients one or another of two equally potent herbs. This book is not as complete as *Dr. Rosenfeld's Guide to Alternative Medicine*, but various chapters tell what works, what doesn't work and what's in the works.

A recent book by Dr. Bernie Siegel *Balanced Healing: Combining modern medicine with safe effective alternative therapies* shows how patients can combine a prescription drug with other therapies such as an herbal supplement, diet and meditation. Most of his extensive book is an alphabetical list of conditions from acne to varicose veins. He discusses the most effective treatment for each. His book includes serious topics such as lowering cholesterol without using statins.

Any of these books is better than searching the Internet, overwhelmed by a plethora of articles, some scientific, some based on testimonials and some blatantly selling a special nostrum. If we believed them all, we could spend much more money than if we relied on expensive prescriptions. Siegel warns never to buy anything sold by multilevel marketing.

The mind-body connection itself can be more important

What we think and how we act can affect the chemicals in our brains and other parts of our bodies. Even 50 years ago, some doctors said that three-fourths of medical conditions such as ulcers, headaches, cancer or heart disease have a psychological component. The connection was usually stress. Both positive and negative emotions can affect the body. Norman Cousins used long daily doses of laughter by watching slap-stick movies to decrease the pain of his ankylosing spondylitis, a serious degenerative disease. Laughter plus high intravenous doses of vitamin C cured him, as reported in *Anatomy of an Illness as Perceived by the Patient.* In the 1980s, after a near fatal heart attack, he wrote *The Healing Heart* and in 1989 *The Biology of Hope* about his cure without drugs.

Detractors say that trying to cure serious disease with positive thinking might keep patients from seeing a doctor, and Cousins' methods could be as harmful as relying on snake oil for cancer. In fact, Patch Adams, a doctor who believes in the therapeutic value of laughter, has dressed up as a snake oil salesman. He uses other outfits including that of a clown with a big red nose.

He doesn't mind looking ridiculous if it brings a laugh to his patients. In his book *Gesundheit,* Adams suggests we all keep a humor journal. We could see for ourselves the relationship of our symptoms with our state of mind. Even a conscious smile when you're sad can make you feel more cheerful as nerves from the muscles in your face affect your brain.

The mind-body connection has been used for cures by a variety of healers over the ages

Dr. Pelletier quotes studies that show religion is a powerful adjunct to healing. In many religions, adherents pray for a person's recovery. Some people visit a holy shrine. As longstanding ailments disappear, they leave their crutches and walk away. Others have been healed by "the laying on of hands" by a preacher at a revival meeting. Faith played a big part in the person's recovery.

For more than 100 years, Christian Science practitioners have helped heal internal maladies. Besides declaring that God is Love, Mary Baker Eddy said that health is like light showing that we are all the children of God. Disease is like darkness, an illusion dispelled by light. Faith or prayer or a change of ideas might allow a person's body to heal itself. Since the body is meant to be well, faith and hope can help heal it. Our bodies have been programmed over eons of time to manifest health if we just provide the means. It's only when purists in various faiths won't accept procedures like vaccinations that problems occur.

For decades in the tiny town of Mosquito, California, a man known as "The Goat Doctor" used methods unrecognized by physicians of his day. He was as skilful as any chiropractor or osteopath in the manipulation of a patient's spine. He recommended healthy diets that included goats' milk and the herbs gathered by his adoptive mother. She had used the powers of nature to cure him of tuberculosis years earlier. They both had a sixth sense that told them what was wrong with the people who came for help. In the book *The Goat Doctor of the Sierras, A Healer of People*, Gloria Hochensmith has collected stories and letters from a few of the thousands who could have given testimonials about their often miraculous healing. People came from Europe and many parts of the U.S. when conventional medical treatments hadn't worked. They came in pain and left healed by an unassuming man who lived simply and wanted to share his gift.

Mind-over-matter can help in weight loss

The program of Dr. Henry Chang in *Weight Lost Forever* starts with a month of trying to maintain your present weight, then a month of a low-calorie diet. A month of maintaining the lost weight alternates with another month of low-calories followed by another of weight maintenance, as long as it takes to reach a realistic goal for the year. He encourages his patients to endure the pangs of the low-calorie diet because it will only last a month at a time. When they see it's possible to then maintain the lower weight, they feel they are in control of their habits and their lives.

Over the centuries, the so-called witches of the Middle Ages and shamans and healers for primitive societies have produced healing by methods that don't seem to have a scientific basis. The main difference from conventional modern medicine is that instead of treating the disease, they treat the whole patient and get to the cause of symptoms by trying to look within a patient's mind, heart and soul. This makes sense; studies of these healers have shown a lowering of patients' blood pressure and an increase of beneficial immune system substances.

Deepak Chopra and other doctors who combine Western and Asian methods of treatment say that besides lowering blood pressure, daily meditation can increase the supply of DHEA, an adrenal hormone that counteracts stress. Dr. Andrew Weil is another healer with a conventional medical education who felt it didn't go far enough. He now incorporates herbal and other ancient remedies in his practice, along with a spiritual outlook.

Treating more than the symptoms

Most alternative healers think that conventional medicine based on complicated surgery and expensive medication still only treats symptoms. We have already shown how the correct diet and adequate exercise can correct many of the rampant metabolic maladies from obesity and diabetes to osteoporosis and heart disease. What can modern medicine do for conditions that seem to have no known cause or definitive cure? These include some forms of cancer, most of the auto-immune diseases and conditions such as fibromyalgia and multiple sclerosis as well as rare ailments such as ankylosing spondylitis. Some type of alternative medicine might better help relieve symptoms so the person can live a more normal life.

Anthropologist Hank Wesselman has studied and participated in shamanic practices in many parts of the world. In primitive societies, people believe in the power of spirits to cure disease and the ability of the shaman to summon them by drumming. Wesselman wants to help Westerners awaken the healing power within themselves by using the primitive method of drumming. He says the frequency of the beat determines the response in the brainwaves of the listener.

Active thinking corresponds to 13 to 15 cycles per second. Three beats per second mirror delta waves of dreaming. Theta waves are stimulated by drumming at four to five beats per second for up to 30 minutes. This rhythm allows a person to remain awake and still reach part of his own unconscious mind. Perhaps it concentrates a person's attention in a way similar to self-hypnosis.

Wesselman says from a holistic viewpoint there are three basic causes of serious disease:

1. Disharmony after a traumatic loss of a loved one, loss of a sense of belonging to a group or a feeling of decreased power. One of these can precede development of cancer.
2. Fear of something real or imagined. This diminishes the action of the immune system, making a person vulnerable to bacteria, viruses and some cancers.
3. "Soul Loss." If complete, it can produce premature death, as with voodoo. Some people can feel a partial loss after early or extended physical, sexual or psychological abuse. Diagnosis

includes blocked memory, apathy and progressive despair that precede a serious physical illness.

Wesselman has seen Western healers cure serious diseases such as cancer or lupus by shamanic methods.

Many primitive people today still think that the casting of evil spells can cause disease. Blaming illness on the malevolent power of a witch doesn't make sense to me. We know the dire consequences of that belief in Salem, Massachusetts. Some sick people try to find a more powerful shaman to counteract the manifestations of witchcraft. Someone who has faith in his healer will recover. If he thinks a witch has more power, he might die. This is especially true of those who believe in voodoo. It's like the old saying "As a man thinks, so is he."

Most healers without a medical background have enough sense to use their methods as an adjunct to conventional medicine, not as a replacement. However, many patients have already been through the medical system without being helped. They are desperate for a cure. Here is where a search for some disharmony in the heart or soul might be effective, even if it can't be based on scientific method. More Americans now accept ancient practices such as acupuncture. These often work even if the explanation doesn't conform to standard anatomy and physiology. Maybe other alternative methods that seem to have no scientific basis stimulate the body to heal itself.

Loving relationships can be very important in both preventing and curing metabolic diseases

Dr. Kenneth Pelletier mentions studies that show the value of faith, hope and forgiveness. He says that anger and hostility can predict heart disease better than the level of cholesterol or blood lipids. In the town of Roseto, Pennsylvania, residents were just as sedentary, overweight and smoked as much as those of surrounding towns in the 1960s and 1970s. The fact that they had half as many heart attacks was attributed to the social support in these close Italian-American families. However, starting in the 1980s, families broke up and sons and daughters moved away.

As the social closeness disappeared heart disease then matched that of other communities.

Dr. Dean Ornish's book *Love and Survival* talks about the power of love to prolong life in the face of adverse risk factors. Though best known for his non-invasive treatment of heart disease, he found that even his program that emphasizes stress reduction was more successful if accompanied by healthy, loving relationships. He says this is much stronger than any placebo effect. He also tells of the healing power of caring for a pet. He mentions a study of persons who had a heart attack. Only 1 percent of those who owned dogs died during the study, while 6.7 percent of those without dogs died in the same period. Dogs give non-judgmental and unconditional love that reduces stress.

Roy told me how a dog had saved his life. He was new to New York and had no close friends at work. The friend whose apartment he shared was on vacation. When Roy's disappointing job looked like it would be eliminated, life seemed bleak and meaningless. He wondered how big a splat he would make if he went to the roof of the building and jumped off. He put on his jacket and started to open the apartment door. Then the little white terrier he was taking care of for his friend came running with the leash in his mouth, eager for a walk. Roy couldn't disappoint him. They went down to the street for a longer walk than usual. Before they returned, Roy bought a newspaper. He scanned the *Help Wanted* ads with the dog snuggled on his lap asleep. Roy knew that he was needed and his feeling of hopelessness lifted.

Loving care makes a great difference

The following anecdote shows the power of a friend's love and care. Louise decided that her multiple sclerosis might never get better and she should get a wheelchair. She lay in bed, hopeless, helpless and depressed. She didn't feel like eating or even drinking water. She forgot that her friend Martha was coming to visit. Martha entered the unlocked door when there was no answer. She was appalled at Louise' dull eyes, dry skin and the peculiar smell of her breath. Martha helped her into her car to go to a hospital emergency room. The doctor said she was very dehydrated and should be admitted to the hospital. She might even need kidney dialysis by Monday morning. Martha convinced him she would help Louise become re-hydrated with plenty of juices over the weekend and then take her to her regular doctor.

The two days of fluids and loving care made a remarkable difference. Louise was no longer lethargic, so Martha took her to an alternative therapist. He prescribed powdered oxidative enzymes to add to her juices and magnetic inserts for her shoes. I wouldn't tell Martha that all enzymes are proteins and proteins are broken down in the digestive system before they have a chance to enter the blood stream to get to body cells. However, the peroxidase and dismutase by mouth wouldn't do any harm. As for the magnetic shoes, I had heard that a doctor at Baylor University used magnets to lessen pain of patients with post-polio syndrome and to decrease numbness in the feet of diabetic patients.

At any rate, Martha's tender loving care and Louise's hope that her body's natural electricity would be augmented by the magnets seemed to relieve her multiple sclerosis. Two months later, Louise felt energetic and did a lot of walking. Was it a spontaneous remission, a placebo effect or mind over matter when Louise felt hope and the love of a friend?

In all cases of chronic disease, it helps to encourage a patient to move. The body senses an increased need and uses its power to heal itself.

Doctors Deepak Chopra and David Simon in the book *Grow Younger, Live Longer* use concepts from Buddhism and ancient Ayurvedic medicine. In a chapter on the power of love, they say personal love is concentrated universal love and every act of love expresses the spirit. They urge you to communicate love in every interaction every day. It helps your immune system and delays aging. You can show love by attentive listening, by expressing appreciation in words, actions and loving touch. They say sexual vitality can be enhanced by some ancient herbs, but subtlety, timing and finesse are more important for a union of the spirit as well as of two bodies. Though this book includes exercises and diet suggestions for a healthy life, the way a person interacts with others seems the most important factor for delaying aging.

Helen had been invited to spend the weekend with a couple who lived in San Francisco. It was late when they met her bus. They showed her their newly renovated house that could have been featured in a magazine. The couple themselves exemplified the beautiful people, with stylish classic clothes on thin bodies. They said they would leave the house early to go to the gym, but she could sleep late. By 9 a.m., Helen was hungry and went down to the stainless steel kitchen eager to make a cup of tea.

When she figured out how to open the cupboard doors she found only packets of herbal tea. An individual package of dry cereal and some skim milk in the refrigerator were the only foods available. Helen was still hungry. There was nothing to read in the living room and the television must have been hidden behind the wood panels for an uncluttered look. The house was cold from the summer fog of San Francisco. Helen finally went for a walk, thinking it was all right to leave the house unlocked in this quiet well-kept neighborhood. She didn't go far in any direction and kept coming back to see if her hosts had returned. They apologized for staying away all morning and took Helen to lunch.

This couple with their emphasis on external appearances should have read *Grow Younger, Live Longer*. They didn't need the parts on diet and exercise but they hadn't demonstrated the most important aspect of the book. They had not shown loving concern for another person.

Look at life from the viewpoint of others

You may know couples where each one feels in the right and won't consider the other person's viewpoint. Some people treat each conversation like a debate. Being right or winning an argument are hollow victories if you lose a friend or make your spouse feel distant. You're not in a Super Bowl game where your value comes from winning. Think of all the friendly tennis games played every weekend. No one always wins and the play is for fun, not for proving who is superior.

The way you think and act can affect both your body and your brain

Dr. Jeff Victoroff in *Saving Your Brain* says mental activity can prevent dementia and other age-related brain diseases. You can form new brain cells as well as make new connections within the brain as long as you live. Whereas new sensory stimuli help a child's brain to develop, an adult must actively use his brain to keep it healthy, making new cells or connections. Passively watching television won't do it. Senior magazines include crossword puzzles to help keep your mind fit. It's good to have an open mind and continue to have a variety of experiences. It's even better to challenge your brain with problem solving or learning a new language. The best way to grow new brain cells is in organizing a skill or information and teaching it to others.

Bob always had a questioning mind. Even as a child he couldn't accept the idea of hellfire and damnation in his fundamentalist religion, though he did marry within his faith. As an adult, he faced myriad problems in World War II. Then he used his inventive mind and a scientific approach in his job dealing with transportation and air pollution. He also studied psychology and a variety of world religions. He accepted new ideas and new experiences. He tried to get his wife interested in going with him to seminars and weekends that celebrated humanism and nature. She held fast to all her old beliefs and didn't want friends outside her church. Her last years were spent in the fog of Alzheimer's disease. He is still going strong despite a stroke. He reads widely, helps others with computer problems and has a wide circle of friends.

Alternative therapies combined with conventional medical treatments can be very effective

You or your healer should provide the conditions that give your body the best chance of recovery. Often simple methods are best. Don't neglect a disease or dysfunction but use the least harmful method to get a cure. Washing a wound with soap and water gets rid of dirt and germs as well as using stronger chemicals such as iodine that can damage cells and delay healing. It's a mistake to rely only on expensive new medical technology. A second cancer or a second heart attack is a wake-up call that just fixing a symptom had not been enough. You must understand the cause of your dysfunction - then aid in the cure. This can be by changing your lifestyle, your way of looking at the world and your interactions with others. Loving another person or even a pet can often prevent disease or help in its cure. Meanwhile, you have relieved stress and strengthened your immune system. The malady will then be less likely to return.

"Age is a state of mind" or "You're as old as you feel" are not idle sayings

A key to a youthful outlook is to be open to new experiences and new ways of looking at old ideas. Your brain isn't hard-wired like a computer. New DNA is formed with new thoughts and actions. Your mind needs to stay just as flexible as your body. As mentioned in an earlier chapter, certain foods, drugs and supplements can change some of the chemicals in your brain. Your body can respond either with destructive behavior or it changes to accept a better lifestyle.

You're never too young to start and never too old to counteract the dysfunctions blamed on aging. The body is meant to be healthy but you have to do the right things to keep it that way. Here, the Golden Mean serves well.

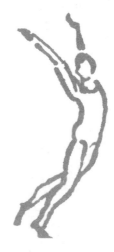

What You Can Do.

- Laugh every day or at least smile. It will brighten the day for all the people you contact. The old-fashioned hymn "Brighten the Corner Where You Are" still rings true.

- Keep track of your moods. See if there's a connection to aches and pains.

- Be open to alternative ways of thinking and alternative therapies. Love and faith can be powerful aids to healing.

- Try to look at every situation from another person's point of view. If there's a conflict try for a win-win result after a compromise.

- Slow down and simplify your life.

- Take time to meditate but don't be rigid. Some days you can only sit quietly for five minutes. Other days you can do the recommended 20 minutes that decreases your blood pressure.

- Welcome the healing power of touching another person or a pet.

- Actively challenge your brain. Work puzzles. Write your Representative in Congress. Learn a new skill and volunteer to teach it to others.

- Instead of trusting only purely physical remedies or only psychological or spiritual ones, aim for a Golden Mean and use both for gaining and maintaining ageless health.

The Cost Of The Status Quo

Factors that seem out of your control can also affect your health.

In this chapter, one section includes anecdotes about toxins. Toxins in the environment and those from manufactured products can produce ailments. Symptoms blamed on aging are caused by chemicals in water, air or household products. Even if these chemicals take a long time to produce symptoms or don't seem to harm everyone, continue to use them at a cost to your present or future health.

Another section tells of increased use of prescription drugs and the rapid rise in prices. Simple methods or supplements might help you as much as either prescription drugs or strong over-the-counter medications. Even if you're not of retirement age, do you think that later you'll be able to afford prescriptions to alleviate the symptoms of aging as well as the metabolic diseases you might be starting to experience now? Can the government or insurance companies afford them?

A section tells of rising health insurance and hospital costs. A family of four might pay more for health coverage than the mortgage on their home. The cost of hospitalization is also rising faster than the inflation rate. The community as a whole will no longer be able to absorb the increased costs for health care.

Take charge of your own health and do everything possible to change your lifestyle so you won't need lots of medications or devices or hospitalizations as you grow older.

17-1 Environmental Toxins
A nutritious diet and adequate exercise might not be enough

for optimum health

We now live in an environmental soup of chemicals, most of which didn't exist 100 years ago. They are in the air, the water the soil and in or on many of our foods. We need to ward off the deleterious effects that come with the promise of "better living through chemistry."

Depression symptoms

Stan should have been very healthy. He had a good diet and took vitamins and other supplements. As an avid surfer, he exercised vigorously. Other activities outside his challenging scientific profession included painting large pictures, some of which were displayed in public buildings. However, he began to feel depressed for no apparent reason. His wife said he was working too hard and that a two-week vacation in Hawaii would do them both good. He jumped at the idea, but for a secret reason.

This would be a chance to end the overpowering depression that was growing worse every day. He would take his surfboard and try the waves on the north shore of Maui. They would be much larger than anything he tried off the coast of California. Starting down one of those waves would be the thrill of a lifetime and the inevitable bone-crushing crash on rocks or coral would end his life in a way that wouldn't jeopardize the life insurance his wife could collect.

The waves at Little Mahaka were indeed magnificent, though not as high as usual, according to the locals. At any rate, Stan went surfing every day. His mental outlook improved along with his skill. By the end of two weeks he agreed with his wife that he was back to normal.

Years later, he analyzed his situation. The months of severe depression had coincided with the period when he made several large acrylic paintings in a small closet alcove of an apartment while waiting for their new house near the beach to be finished. There he would have a studio above the garage for his artistic works. He had chosen to paint with acrylics since unlike oils, they didn't have the toxic fumes of turpentine. The chemicals given off by acrylic paints are more subtle but still dangerous in an enclosed space. He decided to always keep a window open while painting.

I had told Stan about another friend who had less severe symptoms but knew she wasn't up to par. Nancy wondered what was wrong with her. She had no energy, felt depressed and couldn't concentrate. She finally went to her doctor. Too many doctors would have prescribed a tranquilizer and dismissed her as another bored housewife, but he ordered blood tests. They showed a low white cell count, as well as borderline anemia. The liver function tests were somewhat abnormal for no apparent reason. The doctor suggested iron and high potency vitamins.

A few weeks later, I visited Nancy. When I entered the house, I noticed the smell of some chemical but didn't remark about it until she told me about her blood tests. When I asked if she had used a lot of chemical sprays or done any painting in the last few weeks, she said that her monthly termite control service had just been there. I suggested she spend as much time as possible away from the house and cancel the service. Anything strong enough to kill termites or other insects isn't good for humans.

Lawn services that use toxic chemicals can harm your health. Despite the looks of a well-kept golf course, living next to one is now considered dangerous because of the liberal use of both herbicides and insecticides. Is a perfect lawn worth the sacrifice of your health? Remember the long-term effect of Agent Orange on the men who fought in Vietnam? You may be afraid of spiders, but they are beneficial by catching flies and other pesky insects. Most spiders are much less dangerous than any insecticide. We have many of the same cellular enzymes as spiders and insects. Any chemical that can kill them might affect enzymes in your brain, bone marrow, liver or other organs.

Most toxic products sold to the consumer now have warnings

They say, "Use with plenty of ventilation. Be sure this doesn't contact your eyes or skin." Some people anxious to get rid of insects ignore the warnings. I made that mistake when I used

Malathione, an insecticide related to nerve gas. I applied it with a folded rag to the inside of a dresser to get rid of powder-post beetles. I held my breath but didn't wear rubber gloves. I probably absorbed some of the chemical through my skin. By evening, my muscles were very weak and I couldn't lift anything heavy. Even 10 days later, I couldn't take my boys bowling. Weeks later, I went to the doctor when my joints were so sensitive I had to sleep with a piece of foam between the sheet and mattress. Even though I was in my forties, the doctor said this was because I was getting old. I decided the Malathione must have been to blame. My joint pain disappeared after several weeks and I didn't need the mattress pad.

Use the least toxic control for any pest

Never use a stronger solution than recommended of any chemical. Even bleach is more effective against bacteria and molds when diluted. Poison sprays can get into storm drains and kill fish when the run-off enters a river. In our community we can dispose of containers of poison at designated toxic disposal sites. When a fly gets in that I can't get with a fly swatter, I use a spray bottle of water with a drop of dishwashing detergent in it. I crush the disabled fly with a piece of wet paper towel. I use a pump-spray bottle of a simple household cleaner on the lines of ants that sometimes invade the house. This dehydrates their bodies and neutralizes the scent trail that attracts other ants. Instead of using a thin oil spray on scale insects, I found that a solution of household detergent eliminated the scale on my quince tree. Never use aerosol sprays for insects or for household cleaning. Even though they no longer contain Freon gas, you're more likely to inhale aerosol toxins than if you use a pump-spray bottle.

I discovered an easy way to remove paint from the skin. My two-year-old son was in the backyard without his diaper while I was painting a breadbox with an oil-based paint. When a delicate part of his anatomy touched the wet paint, I didn't want to use paint thinner and knew soap and water wouldn't work. I gently applied Vaseline to easily remove all the paint. Petroleum jelly and mineral oil are two benign products from the refining of crude oil and combine with other hydrocarbons. I have also used Vaseline to remove the tar from my hands when I used it on a roof leak in an emergency. I removed the mixture of Vaseline and tar with dry paper towels.

Chemicals can affect any of your organs

Aromatic solvents like benzene and toluene are good for dissolving grease but also react with the fats in your nervous system. Even common liquids such as methyl and isopropyl alcohol or ethylene glycol can be harmful. Ethylene glycol, a common antifreeze in cars, has a sweet taste. You probably know someone who left a pan of ethylene glycol on the floor of his garage when he was changing the antifreeze in his car. His dog lapped up this sweet liquid and got sick or died. Fuels such as gasoline, kerosene and butane can also be dangerous to breathe or get on your skin.

Many industrial and household solvents are damaging, depending on the amount and time you're in contact with them. They include those with chlorine, such as the carbon tetrachloride used in dry cleaning. A man in San Diego who breathed rubber cement all day making wet suits died in his fifties. The chemicals prevented his bone marrow from making either red or white blood cells.

Ethel enjoyed fixing up old houses. She didn't use water-based enamel because it might not last as well. At least she didn't use an alkyd paint. This contains a wood alcohol solvent that can be harmful. (Back during prohibition when unscrupulous sellers diluted their "white lightning made out of corn squeezins" with cheap methyl alcohol, some of their customers went blind.) Ethel really liked the turpentine odor of oil-based paints and used them whenever possible. She mentioned that she had to stop painting after two days because it activated her arthritis. She thought it was because she was using her hand muscles more. I suggested she might be reacting to the turpentine. It doesn't matter that it smelled good; it wasn't good for her. This arthritis was not a natural part of getting old but a reaction to the solvent. I'm even dubious of claims of odorless solvents.

Some products might temporarily inactivate the sensor cells in your nose

I heard of a lawyer who discredited an expert witness who could normally distinguish very faint odors. After the lawyer gave him a whiff of gasoline, the expert couldn't name the rest of the test odors. His ability to smell had been blocked for several minutes. This explanation might apply to the liquid in a small bottle that says on the label: One drop can take away the smell of a skunk. Just because you can't smell them doesn't mean there are no chemical molecules in the air.

I met Jeri on vacation. When I started applying sunscreen, Jeri recoiled and backed away several feet. She explained she was allergic to almost everything. She had been forced to sell her beauty salon when she started to react first to hair sprays, then to all scented products in the shop. Her sensitivity expanded to all air-borne chemicals. She must always carry an inhaler to relieve the sudden wheezing and coughing of asthmatic attacks caused by even small amounts of chemicals.

Avoid man-made substances you can smell or those that produce a shine. The odor of a new carpet is often from formaldehyde molecules being given off. Leave windows open and don't spend much time in the house until the odor is gone. Beware of scented household products and especially of so-called air fresheners. Don't use those you plug in like a night light. They contain para-di-chloro-benzene and are continually adding it to the air. This is the same chemical that kills moths.

Even though modern mothballs are less toxic than the old naphthalene ones, the para-di-chloro-benzene isn't good for you if it can kill moths. The best air freshener is one that actually absorbs odors. It comes as a gel in a conical container. It would be best and just as effective if this had no odor, but the housewife is conditioned to expect a different smell so it is scented. Leave the container open just long enough to absorb offensive odors.

Remember "Mary Hartman" in the satirical sit-com of that name in the 1970s? She was the housewife who worried if her floors were shiny enough or if she should try a different new product. In general, anything that produces a shiny surface probably contains a harmful chemical. If possible, buy flooring that has a permanent finish applied at the factory. I use plain linseed oil on any raw wood to safely produce a nice water-resistant surface.

I have been afflicted with both osteoarthritis and rheumatoid-like arthritis. As mentioned, in the 1990s osteoarthritis began to affect my _right_ knee, the knee immobilized in a long-leg cast many years ago. I can get pain in either knee as a reaction to certain chemicals. The worst was the solvent used in the cement to join PCV pipes. Breathing the vapors has caused pain and swelling, relieved with ibuprofen in a couple of days. Even with low doses of ibuprofen, I take it with food or calcium tablets to lessen the possibility of gastro-intestinal bleeding.

We live with chemicals that didn't exist 100 years ago

More than 170,000 new chemicals have been developed in the past 50 years. Less than half have been tested on healthy adults. Much less is known about possible more devastating effects on the unborn and in young children. Childhood asthma is increasing. Fresno in the Central Valley of California has three times the national rate, as reported in the Autumn, 2002 issue of _Earth Justice_. Chemicals from automobile exhaust in combination with pollens and mold spores can cause allergies in susceptible people. More people, including one out of seven California children, suffer from asthma, only partly controlled by pills and inhalers. You can't quit breathing when you go outside.

Sources of toxins that affect our health might not be obvious

John Harte in _Toxics, A to Z_ tells about multiple sensitivities as well as problems with a variety of single toxins. His Web site links to 259 books and studies on the dangers of modern chemicals. Acrilimide is a chemical that can be formed when substances in potatoes react with high temperature fats to make french fries and potato chips. Since it can cause cancer, the FDA is considering a warning label on these products. It might depend on the fat used. The beef suet formerly used to cook french fries was less likely to form dangerous peroxides at high temperatures than the present polyunsaturated vegetable oils. Maybe it was also less likely to produce acrilimide.

Some cooking utensils might be detrimental to your health

People who were afraid of using fat in cooking started using pans coated with Teflon. This can release perfloric acid, especially in older damaged pans. Some people threw away their aluminum utensils when they heard that Alzheimer's patients have aluminum deposits in their brains. It might be because of faulty aluminum metabolism, not from their pans or anti-acids. However, don't cook an acidic food like tomatoes or sauerkraut in an aluminum pan, since acid does dissolve aluminum. We found that out when we put lemonade mix into an aluminum canteen. Ugh! It tasted poisonous. It's best to use stainless steel cooking utensils or an old-fashioned iron skillet and cook with olive oil.

In the fall of 1989, I moved from San Diego to the hot summers but cold winters of the Sacramento area. It took a while to realize I wasn't just aging fast or was more susceptible to cold weather. A health care advocate for the aged said on the radio, "If you want to know how it feels to be old, put some ball bearings or hard beads into your shoes and try to walk. It hurts the bottoms of your feet so you won't want to walk far." He described how my feet felt when I tried to walk three blocks to the library or even across a parking lot.

What could be causing my problem? I hadn't yet installed dual-paned windows or wall insulation, so I used my fireplace a lot. It had an insert with a fan, so it produced better heat than the inefficient furnace. As a quick way to start fires, I burned the paper towels I used to soak up the fat from the bacon or Spam I ate several times a week as part of a hearty breakfast in the cold house. It wasn't a good idea to eat these meat products because of the nitrites in them. When I stopped eating them, my feet went back to normal and I could walk without pain. I sometimes enjoy bacon or ham at a group meal, but I don't buy products that might contain nitrite preservatives and am better off without them. If I want a breakfast meat, I buy locally grown ground lamb and add chili powder and other spices for the taste of sausage. Sometimes I mix it with a too bland soy-based sausage.

Pregnant women and nursing mothers must be even more careful of toxins

Whereas DDT isn't in breast milk now, PCBs (polychlorinated biphenyls) are an even greater risk to the health and development of infants of nursing mothers. Since 1930, more than 1.25 billion pounds of PCBs have been manufactured. By 1974, The U.S. Department of Interior's Fish and Wildlife Service found PCBs in 90 percent of freshwater fish across the country. A Nutrition Action Newsletter by Marcella Mosher and Greg Moyer tells women to eliminate freshwater fish, cut down on meat and dairy and eat organic produce. Lose weight before you get pregnant to get rid of most of the PCBs in your fat. Maintain your normal body fat during pregnancy since PCBs can cross the placenta. Breast-feed for two days to give your infant the immune protection from your colostrum, and at least two weeks more. If you bottle feed, use organic soy milk or milk from cows or goats that test low in toxins.

Pesticide residue in food is ranked as the number three cause of cancer in the U.S.

The United Farm Workers say migrant field workers are in the most danger. They handle these toxins or are accidentally exposed when insecticides applied by airplanes to another field drift over. Leukemia and lymphatic cancer has increased eight-fold. Debilitating ailments and early death are also higher in migrant farm workers, compared to other groups in the U.S. and other countries. Birth defects in farm workers' children are 13 times higher than in other children. In the U.S., pesticides are used most often on grapes and strawberries. Even if little residue remains on the fruit, there are dire health effects on farm workers. They are exposed to high doses of insecticides and soil fumigants during the whole growth cycle of these crops. Ordinary clothing doesn't protect them.

Contaminants in animal products can be dangerous to consumers. Toxins in animal meat and fat are probably the cause of metabolic disease and cancer, not the fat itself. However, fat gets the blame in scientific articles. Fatty plaque from diseased human arteries should be analyzed for toxins. Since humans have been eating animal fat for millennia, the contaminants in the meat, fat and organs of animals should also be examined. I think the increase in intestinal cancer and cardiovascular disease is being caused by the insecticides, PCBs, dioxins and other chemicals concentrated in this fat, not dietary saturated fat itself. Many pesticides act like weak estrogens and can be cumulative. It is probably one reason more women are suffering from breast cancer and more men have prostate cancer as well as decreased sperm counts.

Water is contaminated by chemicals

Depending on where you live, you might have to drink bottled water or even distilled water because of chemicals in the city water supply. Chlorine is used to kill bacteria in the water, but this reactive ion can combine with industrial contaminants and make them even more toxic.

Pesticides are washed into rivers from cropland. The worst contamination by insecticides, hormones and waste products in many parts of the country comes from factory farms. The natural microorganisms in the storage lagoons can never completely detoxify this wastewater. Is cheaper meat worth the damage to your health and to the environment? Rather than subsidize corn that is used in factory farms, we should encourage the producers of organic meat.

Try to buy locally grown food in season. Pesticide treated food might look attractive but beware. Since most food is now grown on big farms and shipped long distances, it must be treated with chemicals to avoid spoiling. You can see the wax on cucumbers or shiny red apples. Some chemicals that retard spoilage might be less noticeable but more dangerous.

Just because you can buy produce in the winter grown in Mexico or Chile doesn't mean that food is good for you. I would rather buy frozen vegetables grown in California. They are frozen the day they are picked, so aren't contaminated by toxins that retard spoilage. I also buy frozen blackberries, raspberries and blueberries to get these antioxidant-rich berries with fewer pesticides. I buy strawberries in season from a small local grower whose family picks them fresh daily.

Buy at farmers' markets. This produce doesn't have to be picked green to withstand a long journey from the farm to a store, so it tastes better. Lesser amounts or no insecticides are necessary. Since there are fewer trees of any variety in a particular orchard, insect populations aren't liable to grow. Natural predators like birds, ladybugs or a preying mantis can control the few insects.

You can get rid of some pesticides. Soak produce in a solution of a few drops of detergent in a quart of water then rinse it well. If possible, buy apples that aren't shiny with wax. It would be too bad to have to peel off the skin with its vitamins and antioxidants. Some pesticides can't be washed off, according to "Facing the Issue of Pesticide Residues" by Carole Sugarman and a 1987 article by Anne Montgomery. Don't expect the situation to be better today. Dr. Jeff Victoroff in *Saving Your Brain* tells about the dangers to the brain and nervous system of pesticides similar to nerve gas.

Going organic would help consumers, dedicated farmers and the environment

An article by Anne Montgomery, *America's Pesticide Permeated Food*, states that more than 50 years ago, farmers used to lose 7 percent of a crop to insects. Now, even with more and more pesticides, they lose 13 percent. The weedy fence rows between fields encouraged insect-eating birds back then and were good for other wild life. A teenager was able to hunt rabbits or pheasants along the fences. Crop diversity helped as well. Now, with no place for natural predators to live, a single crop planted in giant acreages is much more vulnerable to insects, so more pesticides are used. Most farms are no longer a healthy place to live because of airborne insecticides and herbicides.

Living down-wind from an industrial site is also bad. When I visited the city of Ahmedabad in India, I noticed some areas that reeked of strong odors from industrial chemicals. My body reacted by producing phlegm I had to cough up. This persisted for several days, even after I traveled to other cities. Extra vitamin C and multivitamin tablets helped to counteract the symptoms, but I was glad to leave. Even in America, some industries don't consider the health of those who have to breathe the contaminants they put into the air. Just because people don't have immediate symptoms doesn't mean they aren't harmed.

Do your part to prevent both outdoor and indoor air pollution

Get a modern fireplace insert for much cleaner smoke than an old-fashioned fireplace. Use electric mowers and limb trimmers instead of those with inefficient two-cycle engines. Have a smaller lawn and plant many bushes and trees in your yard to produce oxygen and absorb excess carbon dioxide and the toxins from automobile exhaust. Use potted plants inside the home to help protect you from pollutants in the same way. This is important in tighter, energy-efficient houses. Read the label and think before using any cleaning product. Don't buy it if it's in a spray can that uses a propellant gas; even a manual spray bottle is rarely necessary. A dilute solution of Murphy's Soap on a sponge can clean and shine a variety of surfaces. Mother washed windows with vinegar on a crumpled newspaper. Baking soda can help clean a greasy stove.

Do you want local, state or federal governments to regulate industries so your health doesn't suffer? You can encourage responsible producers by not buying products that harm workers or the environment. You must decide how to change your lifestyle in order to avoid the chemicals our ancestors didn't have to contend with. In all things, prevention is better than cure.

If you can avoid toxins, have a healthy diet and enough exercise, you might not need the drugs and expensive medical procedures that are causing medical costs to skyrocket.

What You Can Do

- Analyze your environment, activities and diet. Could any household products you're using or any foods be related to new symptoms?

- Don't let anyone tell you to expect a lot of aches and pains as you get older. Your body is meant to be healthy. Drugs can relieve symptoms, but you want to get rid of the causes.

- Don't expose yourself to substances that make you feel old before your time.

- Protect your lungs, liver, kidneys, bone marrow and brain by not using toxic chemicals.

- Protect yourself by working outdoors or holding your breath when using solvents and other aromatic chemicals. Wear rubber gloves so the chemicals don't get into your system through the skin. Wearing a mask might protect you from dust but not from chemicals.

- Your liver can neutralize some toxins, but don't depend on it. If you can't avoid being exposed, take extra vitamins, especially C, E & B complex,

- Find alternatives for many household products. If you can smell it, you don't want it. There are too many pollutants you can't avoid. Don't add to their danger

- Your health is more important than shiny floors.

- Soak produce in a dilute detergent solution and then rinse it well to get rid of pesticides.

- Grow your own produce without insecticides.

- Buy organic produce or buy at local farmers' markets. They need fewer pesticides.

- Avoid buying most beef and pork. It was probably grown in a factory farm.

17-2 Prescription Drugs and Possible Alternatives

The 2003 multi-billion dollar Congressional bill for prescription drugs with Medicare will benefit drug companies and seniors with very low incomes. It will have a minor effect on drug costs for others and not cut the overall cost of prescriptions for most Americans. In 2003, according to U.S. Senator Barbara Mikulski of Maryland, Americans spent $184 billion on prescription drugs. In the year ending May, 2002, according to the AARP Bulletin, nine billion more pills were sold. For example, the use of Lipitor has increased tremendously. This is one of the statin drugs that inactivate an enzyme in the liver that makes LDL cholesterol. It used to be given only to the sickest patients with the most atherosclerosis. Now, more than 12 million people take it, despite a cost of $3 per pill.

Some doctors say this is a bargain if it prevents surgery necessary to remove plaque or the by-pass operations on patients with coronary artery disease. In fact many doctors recommend putting people whose cholesterol is only moderately elevated on these drugs as a "preventative measure".

Pills or surgery just alleviate symptoms. You want to remove the causes of disease.

For true prevention, a physician would tell his patients that their liver makes the bad LDL cholesterol from a diet with excessive starches and sugars, especially high-fructose corn syrup. He would warn against the trans fats in margarine and packaged baked goods. As mentioned in the section on cardiovascular disease, trans fats make vessels stiffer and prone to injury. Injuries to the lining of vessels can be caused by nicotine, too high insulin, too much fructose, stress chemicals, certain bacteria and other causes of inflammation. Injuries are then patched by cholesterol. You can prevent a heart attack caused by too much homocysteine by eating a high-fiber diet with plenty of folic acid and vitamins

B-6 and B-12.

The low-fat, high-carbohydrate diet touted by advertisers and many doctors has been causing an epidemic of obesity, diabetes and cardiovascular disease. Despite the fact that eating saturated fat has decreased, heart attacks have increased. As mentioned earlier, the average American consumes yearly 150 pounds of sugar or high-fructose corn syrup, mostly in soft drinks and junk foods. Even teenagers are getting plaque in their arteries from the bad cholesterol made from sugars. Instead of the 8-ounce Coke we drank in the 1950s, a 32-ounce cup of a soft drink is common.

Avoid both too much carbohydrate and too much protein

Eating adequate protein and essential fats decreases abnormal insulin responses. In previous chapters you were alerted to the dangers of eating too much meat. Besides gout, you might increase your risk of cardiovascular disease and cancer from the insecticides in the accompanying fat.

Americans will be paying more for drugs to counteract metabolic diseases. We will pay for drugs directly, through increased health insurance premiums or higher taxes to pay for Medicaid and Medicare. This will cost more billions of dollars as pharmaceutical companies urge doctors to put more patients on their products.

The federal government mandates Medicaid for the indigent, but only pays half of the cost. States are responsible for the rest. In 2002, the cost of Medicaid increased by up to 10 percent. In most states, the Medicaid entitlement is second only to the cost of education, and rising in a time when state budgets are stretched thin. Several states now pay for only the medications on a preference list, usually generic drugs. They no longer blindly fund whatever the doctors, influenced by the pharmaceutical profession, might prescribe.

The use of newer pills caused a price increase for prescriptions of 37 percent in 2001, reversing a trend in the middle 1990s of using more generic drugs. Thoughtful doctors wonder if Vioxx and Celebrex, at $2 a pill, are really better for their arthritis patients than over-the-counter ibuprofen. In fact, news reports said that Vioxx had been withdrawn in September, 2004, because of heart attacks in many users. However, with the slick advertisements in magazines and television directing patients to ask for exciting new drugs, many physicians respond. The colorful ads have a multibillion dollar effect.

It is not inevitable to get arthritis as you get older and have to take medications for it

As I wrote earlier, I had been taking six to 10 ibuprofen pills a day for arthritis in my knees and still had to use a crutch or cane to get around. I even had crutches by my bed so I could get up at night. Sometimes, in order to sleep, I put a sock and leg-warmer on my right leg. I could then put my leg, bent at a right angle outside the covers with the foot resting on the floor. Since I could no longer ride a bicycle, I walked wearing a knee brace and used a cane for a round trip of a mile-and-a-half a couple times a week. I went on Audubon bird-watching trips as well, even though it hurt to bend my knee getting in and out of a car. As mentioned in another chapter, when I heard Dr. Andrew Weil tell how ginger root can act on the same body chemicals as do the non steroid pain-killers in relieving the pain and inflammation of arthritis, I started using it in cooking every day. After a while, I used only one or two ibuprofen a week, if I had done some strenuous hiking.

Physicians suggest pills and tell you to use your joints if you have arthritis. They should emphasize that the purpose of anti-pain pills, whether aspirin, Tylenol or other medication is to enable you to **use your joints**, not just to feel better while sitting around. Tylenol won't erode your stomach, but it only helps with pain. Aspirin, naproxen and ibuprofen decrease inflammation as well as relieve pain. However, they have all caused erosions or bleeding of the gastro-intestinal tract in some people. Ginger doesn't have the potentially dangerous side-effects of these pain medicines.

Some people say taking chondroitin and glucosamine pills should help arthritis since they are constituents of cartilage. To me, that's as simplistic as saying to eat Jell-O to help your nails since it's made from the hoofs of animals. A more complete protein helps your nails better than gelatin. Can either chondroitin or glucosamine escape being broken down during digestion? I don't know of studies using radioactive tagged molecules showing that either the glucosamine or chondroitin you take by mouth becomes the cartilage in your joints. Maybe these substances act on other chemicals associated with inflammation. If they work for you, they are better than dangerous pain pills.

Other inflammatory conditions can be helped by methods that don't require pills

Miriam, who works in a small office, said that she no longer has the symptoms of carpal tunnel syndrome. After she changed her diet and started exercising, the pain went away. She thinks that shifting gears or putting on the brakes while riding her bicycle is the major factor in healing her wrist. Those movements were intermittent and allowed periods of rest. Also she modified the time she spent at each office task. This seems more sensible than just taking pain pills.

As a novice tennis player, striving to improve, I was dismayed when my right elbow hurt so much I couldn't even lift a cup of coffee. Someone said to get rid of the tendonitis of "tennis elbow" by first using ice, then keeping the elbow warm. When I got back to playing, I always used an elbow warmer made from the cuffs of socks. Black was best because it absorbed sunlight.

Any inflammation of connective tissue can be painful, but the worst was a bursitis of my shoulder blade, caused by a cold wind on my back when I was digging in the garden just before a week-long camping trip in Mexico. When I was lying down and the shoulder blade was warm, it was all right. If I tried to turn over and especially if I tried to sit up, the pain was excruciating. When we got back to civilization, the doctor gave me Motrin (a high dosage ibuprofen) and scheduled several sessions of ultra-sound, a form of deep heat. From then on, I avoid cold air and wear a sweater in the summer when I enter a building with air-conditioning. Prevention is better than cure.

Besides the cost of prescription drugs, their overuse can harm your health

According to an article in the AARP Bulletin of November 2003, as more people take more drugs for more conditions, adverse reactions become a serious health threat. Older people have two to three times as many reactions as younger people. They might not absorb drugs as well or have greater side effects. Pharmacy alerts of potential problems for patients over 65 increased to 7.9 million in 2002. Since many elderly take more than eight different medications, drug interactions are liable to cause problems. Also, 20 percent of older people take prescription medications that can impair their balance or cause mental confusion. This can lead to a fall and a broken bone.

Consider simple remedies before you rush to a doctor, clinic or emergency room. There might be a simple remedy to take care of temporary pain or discomfort. Even if a third party is paying the bill, all patients will pay more in higher premiums later. You might try heat or cold or heed the old advice: "Take two aspirin and call me in the morning." Of course, if pain is severe and persistent or accompanied by a fever, you should at least talk to an advice nurse.

When you see a doctor, ask whether you really need an expensive medicine or if a generic or some simple procedure is just as good. Many seniors now pay more for pills than for food every month. By eating a more healthful diet, they might not need any drug. People eating the Atkins diet say they no longer need insulin for type II diabetes. However, they might have other problems later.

More isn't better, whether applied to food, supplements or prescription drugs

Try to use only the amount that relieves your symptoms. As

mentioned earlier, both Schwarzbein and Ross individualize diets to their patients so they no longer need drugs and supplements. The human body is complex, so each cell makes what it is programmed to do as long as it gets essential amino acids, essential fats and certain vitamins in a complete, healthy diet accompanied by adequate exercise.

Don't be swayed by colorful advertisements, Internet testimonials, radio hucksters or even what your doctor says. Doctors learn about new medicines from pharmaceutical representatives who give them brochures and free pills. The media is dependent on advertisers. Notice how many ads suggest you ask your doctor for a certain pill. Most of these just treat symptoms. If you continue with the lifestyle that causes those symptoms, you'll be more dependent on prescriptions.

Take charge of your own health. Learn as much as you can and decide what makes sense over the long-term. You can't go wrong by eating natural foods, increasing exercise and improving relationships with your family and others. Believe in the power of the body to heal itself.

You can take care of your health. Then you won't need a lot of prescriptions and expensive procedures. You won't have to wonder if your insurance company or a government agency will pay your medical bills. You won't have to decide whether to spend $90 or more for *each* of several prescriptions every month or buy groceries and pay the utility bill with the money. You won't have to feel like a victim. The sooner you start, the healthier you will be. You can avoid debilitating aging using the Golden Mean in diet, exercise, mental outlook and lifestyle.

17-3 Health Insurance, Hospitalization and Immunity

Legislation that purports to help seniors with costs of medications and hospitalization in reality helps pharmaceutical companies and the manufacturers of ever more complex medical machines or purveyors of new procedures.

Seniors stay in hospitals longer and take more medication

The burgeoning cost of Medicare should concern the estimated 77 million aging Baby Boomers and both political parties. The purpose of an HMO (health maintenance organization) is to promote healthy habits throughout life. Besides pamphlets, classes and seminars, some HMOs have decreased the case loads of many of their doctors, allowing them more time with patients to emphasize prevention, You shouldn't have to take it easy to avoid serious mishaps or disease. A healthy person has a good heart and lungs, strong bones, flexibility, good muscle tone and good balance. If you take the time and effort to get these, you won't end up in a hospital with a fractured hip, a heart attack, a stroke or other serious condition. You can get healthy and stay healthy. It's not too late to try.

Forty-three million Americans don't have any health insurance

They work hard for small employers who are barely able to pay their wages, much less pay for health costs. Premiums for this insurance are spiraling up every year. Most strikes of union workers in 2003 and 2004 have been because employers were no longer going to provide free or low-cost health insurance. Workers in privileged industries only have to pay a minor part of the bill themselves.

The average premium had gone up 14 percent in 2003, the third year of increases greater than 10 percent. It would do no good if new laws let you deduct your health insurance costs or get a credit on your taxes if your taxable income is too low. Minimum wage workers pay more in Social Security than income taxes. Some big employers give good health insurance benefits to regular workers, but make sure that a large number of their employees are part-time or temporary so not eligible for benefits. As insurance premiums keep rising, a smaller proportion of workers will be full-time. Those with higher salaries might work more than 40 hours a week. If they're called independent contractors they have to pay their own health costs.

The working poor

Nicholas is one of the uninsured, a member of the working poor. Though trained as a journalist, he doesn't have a regular job. He writes plays and makes documentaries in a college community. In order to live, he does manual labor for small employers. This includes clearing land, pruning trees or doing landscaping on a per job basis. He usually has time for intellectual pursuits, but some days he works so hard he goes to bed right after supper. He has never had health insurance and hasn't needed it because of his active lifestyle and healthy diet.

Nicholas didn't consider possible accidents. While walking on a windswept bluff above the ocean near San Louis Obispo, he suddenly felt a sharp pain in his ankle. As he jerked back, he saw the thick body of a rattlesnake slithering into the brush. It took more than an hour for him to limp back to the road and get a friend to drive him to the nearest hospital. He was admitted, given anti-venom and an intravenous drip to stabilize his condition. The doctor told him he got the anti-venom within the four-hour window that ensures recovery. *Croatalus viridens* snakes are common along the coast. He said they treat six or seven cases a year and always have anti-venom on hand. Four days later, Nicholas was driven several hundred miles home to Santa Cruz, where he was admitted to the local hospital for follow-up care.

He was back to normal within a couple of weeks, but was aghast at the medical bill of more than $66,000. At least he had been treated as an emergency without anyone first asking about insurance. There's no way he can pay that bill with his income. If he were indigent, he would be eligible for Medicaid. As a member of the working poor who doesn't even own a car, he could not afford the monthly premiums for health insurance.

In Northern California, a single person in his fifties can pay $260 a month if enrolled in a Kaiser Permanente Personal Advantage plan in 2003. Blue Cross/Blue Shield or other plans would probably be similar. It's no wonder that having high medical bills is a major reason for declaring bankruptcy by people with low to moderate incomes, according to numerous sources on network television or the radio.

Health insurance plans change yearly, and costs will go up

You may be lucky and have a good insurance plan, but it's better to stay healthy. Wouldn't you rather stay out of the hospital and not need a lot of medications? I'm reminded of a woman in the 1940s who said she wasn't worried about her children contracting polio from swimming in the city pool because the family had bought polio insurance.

Of course, insurance doesn't magically prevent disease. It just decreases the financial burden. Taking 13 percent more from a retired person's Social Security benefit for Medicare won't cover increasing costs. The average person, whether working or retired, will pay more in premiums with higher deductibles or pay higher taxes to cover health care as he ages. Medicare will be bankrupt if this trend of ever-increasing medical costs is not reversed.

Medical and hospital bills have increased much faster than inflation in the last 20 years. In the 1980s, I was in a strange city attending a convention when I noticed pus around a sliver in my finger, an obvious infection. I called a nearby doctor's office and learned the fee would have been a minimum of $75. An emergency room visit would have cost twice as much. (Today's costs might be four or five times higher.) So I bought Epsom salts at a drug store and soaked the finger in a strong solution that evening to draw out the sliver and the pus. The finger was back to normal the next morning. Being in good health helped rapid healing at minimum cost.

Heart disease is the leading cause of death in the U.S.

More women are suffering heart attacks than before, just like men. In the past, women often weren't diagnosed. Doctors thought that natural estrogen in pre-menopausal women and hormone replacement after menopause prevented heart attacks. As more women smoke, they succumb to the same effect of nicotine that causes small arteries in the heart to clamp down, as well as a faster heart rate and higher blood pressure. Young women who smoked to stay thin would "worry about their hearts tomorrow." Tomorrow has arrived for many or them.

Despite extensive expensive surgery you can have a second heart attack

Estimates of the cost of cardiovascular disease range from $78 billion to $94 billion annually. It costs $30,000 or more for bypass surgery to replace clogged coronary arteries. Balloon angioplasty, where a tube is passed through the arteries to flatten out the plaque, is simpler but costs about $7,000. Neither procedure gets to the causes of heart disease and must be redone a few years or even a few months later as more fatty plaque accumulates. Dr. Ornish's lifestyle changes are as effective as surgery and more long-lasting. His patients have improved their basic physiology.

Taking more medications to treat the symptoms isn't a safe quick fix to avoid surgery

Kenneth Pelletier's book, *The Best Alternative Medicine* says there are more than 100,000 deaths a year associated with prescriptions and over-the-counter drugs. The cholesterol-lowering drug Baycol was withdrawn because of deaths. Other "statin-type" drugs are best used only for genetic high cholesterol. As shown earlier, most people can raise HDL cholesterol with exercise and lower LDL cholesterol by avoiding sugars that the liver makes into cholesterol and fat.

Many Americans are so afraid of heart disease they want the most advanced treatment. The CBS program *60 Minutes*, aired February 16, 2003, showed how a greedy cardiologist was able to dupe patients into undergoing unnecessary coronary bypass surgery. Doctors, the hospital and its corporate owner made a lot of money from insurance companies and Medicare by doing procedures that potentially harmed normal patients. This type of fraud raises all health insurance premiums.

Prevention is better than cure for most medical conditions

Buying a $100 mattress pad cover can prevent asthmatic attacks at night in persons allergic to dust mites in the mattress. A hospital stay for acute asthma might cost from $1,000 to $10,000, according to a study by CalPERS (a California Public Employees health plan). Any HMO should see the financial benefit of the mattress pad in preventing a costly hospital admission. Dust mites are not a new problem.

Back in the 1940s, my father suffered from allergic rhinitis. Skin tests showed the most reactive allergen was household dust (probably from dust mites) that couldn't be avoided. He finally had an operation to cut away the swollen tissues inside his nose so he could breathe. Surgery is always a radical solution to a problem. Joan showed me an air-cleansing unit she uses in her home. She also has a vacuum cleaner that traps dust in water that can be discarded.

Clean indoor air is a start, but more people get asthma from outdoor air. If everyone used a carpool or other transportation two or three days a week or bought a hybrid car, pollution could be cut in half. Would automobile users be willing to pay a health tax added to the cost of gasoline to help pay for the damage their internal combustion engines are causing? People might cut down on unnecessary driving. Funds from the tax might provide health insurance for the working poor and prevent more hospitals from closing due to inadequate funding.

Hospitals have the mystique of being temples of healing with space-age gadgets

But many hospitals don't live up to our expectations. They can be harmful to your health. Hospitals are once again dangerous places, with the rise of antibiotic-resistant bacteria causing untreatable infections and the smaller staffs prevalent in today's cost-conscious medical community. Two million patients acquire infections in hospitals per year according to the U.S. Centers for Disease Control and Prevention as reported in the November 2004 issue of the AARP *Bulletin.* Many widely reported studies state that 35 percent of surgical hospital deaths are caused by these infections. Many hospitals are becoming reservoirs of antibiotic-resistant bacteria. Hospitals might have to go back to chemical sterilization of everything that can't be treated by pressurized steam.

In the first half of the twentieth century, hospitals were safe but reeked of the carbolic acid used to kill all bacteria. Disposable needles were introduced in the 1950s after we learned that viruses, such as those causing hepatitis, can survive the steam of an autoclave. Penicillin and other antibiotics introduced in the 1940s and 1950s killed most disease bacteria.

This golden age of combating disease didn't last. Antibiotics were over-used. As early as the 1950s, broad spectrum antibiotics were fed to animals to speed up their growth. Cows were given penicillin to prevent udder infections. Veal animals needed even more antibiotics because they must be anemic to keep their flesh white. Meanwhile, doctors prescribed antibiotics for virus diseases even though they didn't work. Overuse caused mutation of bacteria and the remaining super-bacteria flourished. Only one or two antibiotics can now kill staphylococci. It's hard for researchers to keep ahead of resistant strains of bacteria as well as combat new microbes from other parts of the world that travel with the speed of airliners. Get healthy so you can stay out of hospitals.

A competent nursing staff can help make a hospital stay safer, but a shortage of nurses is already evident. An article in the May 2003 AARP *Bulletin* tells of two studies on the importance of nurses. The Harvard School of Public Health in a review of 6 million patients in U.S. hospitals concluded that death from complications increased in hospitals with fewer registered nurses. A University of Pennsylvania study showed that a patient's risk of death rose 7 percent with every patient over four that a nurse had to care for. Unless more nurses are trained and the burn-out rate of 20 percent is stemmed, it will be worse. Licensed vocational nurses and nurses' aides can do routine hospital tasks but it takes someone with more education to assess changes in a patient's condition and know when to alert a physician.

Your best defense against disease is keeping your immune system healthy

In the early Twentieth Century, doctors realized that people living in overcrowded slums or in polluted mining and factory towns were more likely to get tuberculosis and die from it than those in small farming communities. Fresh air, along with simple healthy food became the standard treatment for tuberculosis. Those with money went to fancy spas in Switzerland like the one described in Thomas Mann's *The Magic Mountain*. Those with modest means went to sanatoriums where most activities were held outdoors. I saw a picture of children sitting at school desks out in a field, wearing coats and scarves to keep warm. With a healthy diet and fresh air, their bodies could surround the tuberculosis bacteria with calcium and keep these microbes inactive. Even after anti-tuberculosis drugs were used in the 1950s, some doctors said the disease was related to the patients' inadequate immune systems.

Now, 50 years later, illegal immigrants in sweat-shops or crowded farm labor camps are getting and spreading tuberculosis. A big problem with anti-TB drugs is they must be taken daily without fail. If a patient's sputum still tests positive, another drug must be used against the probable resistant microbes. Our public health system can't give these workers the long-term drugs they need and no one monitors their housing. If part of the population is carrying a contagious disease, even people in better parts of town are in danger. The U.S. Public Health Service must protect the whole population, including undocumented workers. Cutting funds to save tax dollars or restricting treatment to select groups is short-sighted. For a country to be strong, everyone living there must be healthy.

Antiseptics aren't the answer

Bacteria and viruses can spread anywhere. Wiping off door-knobs won't help you if a germ is in the air. Several years ago, bacteria in the ventilating system of a building infected people with Legionnaires' disease. It is counterproductive to use a mouthwash that kills all bacteria or a strong antiseptic on your skin or to wash all surfaces in your home with a germ-killing solution. You should keep the normal friendly bacteria in and on your body to crowd out dangerous ones and to prevent the growth of yeasts and molds. It takes stronger chemicals to treat an infection caused by these organisms. Veterans of Pacific wars got what was called "jungle rot" from these yeasts and molds.

A too-sterile environment can be detrimental. In the 1930s and 1940s, many adults got polio because in childhood their mothers tried to keep them germ free. Since they never had a mild form of the disease, they did not produce antibodies that would have protected them from later infection with the polio virus. Warding off viruses depends on your immune system. Limited contact with most infectious agents helps build your body's defenses. Some, like the AIDs virus, are exceptions.

No research has confirmed the following anecdote, but it might help you. When my older son was in kindergarten, he came home one afternoon feeling weak and tired. Thinking he might be getting a cold, I gave him 250 mg. of vitamin C and put him to bed. No cold developed. A few months later, he and his younger brother spent the weekend with playmates who later developed chicken pox. Only my younger son soon had the typical rash of that disease. The older one never showed any symptoms. Maybe he had been exposed to chicken pox at school. Perhaps vitamin C had prevented it from developing but allowed his immune system to produce antibodies to the virus.

Pollutants in the environment can affect your immune system. The section on toxins told of other ways they can harm your body. The combination of a chemical plus the presence of pollen or mold spores can cause your immune system to over-react and produce an allergy. Sometimes toxins poison the liver or bone marrow so you can't make antibodies or enough white blood cells to attack bacteria or viruses. Insecticides are some of the worst offenders.

You must build a healthy immune system. You will be able to cope with bacteria, viruses and pollutants. It will keep you out of hospitals.

Food for thought:

- Health insurance is necessary for emergencies, even for the healthy.
- The U.S. needs a universal medical care system.
- Health problems of the least fortunate can affect everyone.

Our present health system is not addressing these problems. As the richest country on earth we can't afford to continue with the status quo. Write your Representative in Congress or your newspaper. Talk with your health provider, your church or your social groups.

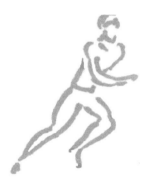

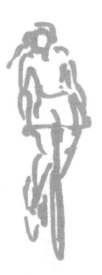

What You Can Do:

- Your best hope against any kind of disease is to keep your immune system strong by diet, exercise and avoiding pollutants and other toxins.

- You might need extra vitamins, minerals and antioxidants.

- Exercise should be adequate but not excessive.

- If you come down with a virus, don't tough it out and go to work anyway. Your co-workers will appreciate your not spreading your germs in the early, most infectious stage.

- Drink plenty of liquids and get some bed rest. The average American needs more sleep anyway. Sleep deprivation can harm your immune system.

- Though controversial, 2 to 3 grams of vitamin C in divided doses while you're home might help your body cope with most virus diseases.

- Unless you have a special reason not to be immunized, take the standard shots for bacterial and virus diseases. More than 80 percent of the population must be vaccinated to make an epidemic unlikely.

- Vote for measures that provide routine health care for the uninsured. You're paying for it already in higher premiums when they have to go to emergency rooms for treatment.

- Sitting around popping the latest pills either for a metabolic condition or an infectious disease is not as effective as staying healthy.

- Prevention is better than cure and much less expensive.

Your Final Years

Most of us will live well beyond the three-score years and ten predicted when Social Security was introduced. Comparisons with other countries are misleading. When they say the life expectancy in Third World countries is 45, while ours is 77 years, it refers to the life expectancy at birth. Many babies and young children die in countries with inadequate sanitation but anyone who survives to adulthood can live as long as we do.

It is heartening that many seniors delay retirement, start a new career or get active in volunteer work. These are the healthy ones. However, some of them could not function without taking a lot of pills.

Everyone hopes to live a long healthy life and die in their sleep after a brief mild illness that provides just enough time to straighten out their affairs and say good-bye to loved ones at the bedside. However, we all know people who ended up differently. Sometimes a long serious illness puts someone in the hospital on life support with a needle in a vein and tubes in various body orifices. The person's body is alive, but he can't communicate with anyone, and loved ones can only hold his hand and listen to the rhythm of the machines. Do you want to end that way?

Most deaths can be postponed if you take care of your health

Dr. Kenneth Pelletier studied the difference between leading causes of death reported in autopsies and actual causes of death. In one typical year, three top diagnoses were heart disease at 750,000; cancer at 505,000; and stroke at 144,000. The three top actual causes of death were tobacco at 400,000; [faulty] diet and inactivity, 300,000; and alcohol, 100,000. Other causes were less than 92,000. HIV took 25,000 lives and illegal drugs killed 20,000. The point is that most deaths can be postponed if you take care of your health.

Before the twentieth century, hospitals were dangerous places and many patients sent there died. Now that fewer antibiotics are effective, hospitals are again unsafe. No matter how much technology advances, you're better off staying healthy. Then you won't need to go to a hospital or have a lingering semi-life in a nursing home.

If you stay healthy, you will be able to choose how you spend your final years, whether traveling, enjoying the arts or learning new skills. You won't be afraid of falling and can choose to be independent.

18-1 Falls can occur as you age, but they need not be serious

Janice, in her early sixties, fell when she stepped off a curb in Chicago. When she realized she had hurt her wrist, she had a taxi driver take her to the nearest hospital. First, the admissions clerk asked about her health insurance. With her HMO card she could get emergency treatment outside of her home city. She was directed to the benches outside the emergency room.

Janice waited with scores of others, including many a mother trying to comfort a sick child and keep her other children out of trouble. A sign on the wall said patients might be seen out of turn. First, victims of gunshot wounds, auto accidents, possible heart attacks and a thin elderly woman gasping for breath, were sent to be examined by interns in tiny curtained cubicles.

After a three-hour wait, a doctor asked Janice to try to move her fingers. He felt her throbbing arm and sent her to X-ray for another long wait. The x-ray showed that both bones in her forearm had been broken. Another young doctor applied a plaster cast she was to keep on for six weeks. It had now been more than five hours since her accident. Janice wondered why a simple fall caused the broken bones. She had given up cigarettes long before smoking was seen as one cause of osteoporosis. She didn't drink much coffee; she had a decent diet with vegetables and meat. She did enjoy one or two glasses of wine a day and never passed up a dessert.

Janice was married in the 1950s when women were encouraged to be feminine and not use their muscles. It was the man's job to mow the lawn, take out the trash, move a typewriter or sewing machine for his wife or do other tasks requiring even moderate lifting. After her children entered pre-school, she didn't even carry them around. A gradual loss of bone, along with the weakening of the muscles in her upper body began in her mid-thirties and continued. She didn't realize that meat and phosphates in soft drinks might deplete calcium more than caffeine.

In contrast to Janice's short fall, I had two severe falls in my mid-sixties but didn't break any bones. On one occasion, I was on a hike in the sierra trying to catch up with younger members of the group. We were boulder-hopping near a ridge above a sheer cliff overlooking a lake. One of the rocks I stepped on shifted, causing me to fall, face-forward onto a stable granite slab. I took most of my weight with my right hand. This hand was painfully bruised but I broke no bones. It took a few weeks before I could use the hand for unscrewing the tight lid of a jar, but ordinary daily activities were never a problem. For a couple of years in cold damp weather, my right wrist hurt but never enough to limit its use.

A few years ago I visited my son and his active octogenarian landlady, Hilda. She said she was recovering from a fall a few months before and had just stopped using a sling for her right arm.

"After falling, I thought it was just a sprain and I didn't know where to go since the Community Hospital had closed," Hilda told me. "A week or two later, I went to a friend's Medicare doctor. He said the two bones in my forearm weren't lined up right so he would have to break them and reset them. It would take longer before I could use my arm. When the nurse told me they didn't take Medicare any more, I cancelled the appointment. It is hard to twist my wrist but I can do almost everything I need to do. I'm glad I didn't have it re-broken and re-set."

I noticed that Hilda's right forearm and wrist looked much larger than the left and seemed awkward and board-like. I remarked, "If you had been examined the day you fell, you would have full use of the wrist by now."

"This didn't seem as serious as a fall I had about a dozen years ago," Hilda continued. "I caught all my weight on my right hand. That night my arm started to hurt. When it got black and blue and swollen the next day, I went to the hospital emergency room. The young doctor saw only minor cracks in the bones of my hand on the x-ray. He wrapped my arm and hand and suggested ice packs and Tylenol. Later, a senior doctor reviewed the x-ray and called to tell me my elbow was dislocated and to come in right away to have it reset. I told him I would wait until the swelling went down. I never did go in and the arm got back to normal. I expect this will get better, too."

When I visited Hilda a couple of years later soon after her 89th birthday, I looked at her wrist. The right wrist and forearm now looked similar to the left and she was peeling potatoes with ease. The excess calcium deposits that had formed around the bones as they were healing must have been absorbed. The bones themselves had been gradually remodeled with use and returned to their normal separate functions.

This reminded me of my own experience when I broke both bones in the lower part of my right leg after falling off a glacier many years ago. The surgeon used two screws to hold the pieces of the tibia (shin-bone) together. He ignored the small bone beside it, the completely fragmented fibula. However, an x-ray taken many years later showed I had a fully functioning fibula formed from the splinters. Bones are living tissue, shaped by the stresses exerted by the attached muscles. Some healers call this the wisdom of the body.

Bone density affects the outcome of a fall

The typical osteoporosis victim is usually thin. She often eats a limited, low-protein diet. When one friend learned her bones were becoming too thin, she didn't want to take hormones or Fosamax to prevent further loss of calcium. She gave up coffee, tea and alcohol and became a vegan vegetarian. Time will tell if she is absorbing and keeping enough calcium in her body.

Unfortunately, many vegans eat too little good-quality protein. Bone has a matrix of protein on which the calcium salts are deposited. On the other hand, eating too much meat can deplete calcium because its excess phosphorus combines with calcium and goes out in the urine. This is not true of eggs, which have a good ratio of phosphorus and calcium.

Another thin acquaintance doesn't want to forego her two glasses of wine a day, so she takes calcium pills and exercises two or three hours a day, working on machines in a gym, and attending classes in yoga and dance exercise.

You don't have to go to either of these extremes of diet or exercise. Hilda has been riding a bicycle since her adolescence in England. She helped in her husband's landscaping business and still does her own gardening. She eats a good mixed diet, including meat and plenty of green vegetables. She drinks strong tea and occasionally has wine. She has taken bone meal tablets for many years. She thus gets calcium and magnesium and enough protein for good bones.

As you exercise more and eat a healthy diet, you will feel more confident that a fall might not result in a broken bone. Even if you do break a bone, you will heal readily. You won't be like some frail elderly people who break a hip just turning over in bed. Hip-bone replacement surgery might not even work if your pelvic bone is too weak from loss of calcium. This is another case where you shouldn't want to be thin. You want to strive to be healthy so a fall won't put you in a wheelchair for the rest of your life. You want to be able to live a normal life.

18-2 Can you stay in your home?

Have you considered what your final years will be like? The habits you form in your twenties and thirties or changes you make in the following decades will determine if you barely exist or live a zestful life. Added years can provide new experiences among new friends and continued connection with family and old friends. You don't have to worry about ending up in a nursing home if you take care of your health and your relationships. Even those who choose to live alone can feel they're doing more than just marking time in their later years.

If you're not healthy, living alone can be dangerous

Consider this incident in the last year of life of a 77-year-old woman described below, as if from her viewpoint:

Cora felt a cold wind on her face and opened her eyes. She saw the light from the naked bulb above her. She realized she was lying on the basement floor with her left leg folded under her right. The leg hurt and she couldn't get it out from under the other one. It hurt to move her right leg because of arthritis in the knee. She always wore an elastic knee brace when she went shopping, but hadn't thought she would need it until she was half-way down the steep steps from the back porch to the basement. By leaning on the railing she went down the stairs, but didn't remember falling.

She rolled from side to side, but it hurt her lower back. She struggled, rested and tried again. Finally both legs were straight in front of her. She would then have to roll on to her abdomen and push with her hands to get one knee under her and use the strongest leg to stand up. Not having eaten in two days made her weak and faint. She decided to rest a few minutes before trying to get up.

What a week it had been – snow or cold wind every day. She couldn't go shopping because of the weather, even though the grocery store was only two blocks away. Unwilling to chance slipping on the icy sidewalks, she had stayed inside, using up the food in the kitchen cupboard. Her favorite meal now was creamed corn with finely ground nuts and chunks of a chocolate bar. Another was hot cinnamon toast spread with mashed ripe bananas. She could almost smell it.

She thought she would rest some more then get up and rummage through the storage pantry for canned fruit or vegetables that wouldn't bother her dentures. Maybe some of the spaghetti bought when her deceased husband had found a bargain didn't contain meat sauce. For the past 35 years she had been a vegetarian. The main thing she remembered from her college course in home economics was that meat contained "awful amino acids that turned into urea." [As I mentioned in another chapter, amino acids are essential for building new body proteins and enzymes. When amino acids are metabolized as carbohydrates, urea is a normal by-product.]

The next thing she knew, two strong young men were lifting her and carrying her to her bedroom. She heard the voice of a neighbor, Mrs. Lawson, "Are you all right? We noticed the basement light was on all night so we thought we better check."

Mr. Lawson added, "When you didn't answer the front door I went around back and down the open cellar door. After I saw you lying there, I called the fire department. My wife called your daughter Ruth long distance. She said she would fly out right away."

The paramedics meanwhile were taking Cora's vital signs. "Your pulse is very slow and your temperature is in the low 90s. You're lucky you had such good neighbors. They called us just in time. It's still below zero outside." Cora couldn't respond to any of the voices but relaxed as they took her to the community hospital in this northern Colorado town.

By the time her daughter arrived from the East Coast, Cora was sitting up. Ruth heard her tell the nurse, "I feel fine and want to go home. It's too expensive to stay in a hospital anyway."

The doctor came by on his morning rounds. "I'm glad you're here. When I checked your mother yesterday, I found no evidence of a stroke or injury and no sign of diabetes to explain why she passed out. She's a little anemic but since you're here, she can go home now."

Ruth asked later, "Don't you have Medicare, Mom? If not, we better see that you get enrolled. When Dad died six years ago, I should have asked you then. I'll see about getting you the *Meals on Wheels* program. It can be vegetarian but you should get at least one hot meal a day. I'll have a visiting nurse stop by every few days as well."

Cora didn't object to these arrangements but cancelled them when Ruth left. She was fiercely independent and wary of strangers in her home.

You need information to stay healthy on your own

Let's analyze this episode that involved my mother and older sister. It could be typical of many older women living alone. If you are still able to make rational decisions, you might prevent your own life-threatening event. Cora didn't believe in doctors, but she didn't have the right information to stay healthy on her own. She could have had a balanced diet with adequate protein from eggs, cheese or beans if she didn't want meat. In the 1970s, there wasn't the range of soy-bean products that provide all the essential amino acids contained in meat. Today's seniors should be able to have a healthy diet, but like most Americans, many are buying packaged manufactured foods instead of fruit, vegetables and good protein sources. It's little better than the tea and toast that many elderly women used to subsist upon.

In medical school, I saw many older patients with a variety of symptoms for which they received 10 to 15 prescriptions at the clinics in the county hospital. We weren't taught to even ask about diet. Medicine concentrated on relieving symptoms. One medical resident surprised me with a suggestion for the weak old lady I had examined. He said she might cure most of her complaints by taking a tablespoon of brewers' yeast stirred into water or broth morning and evening. It didn't sound scientific, but was more sensible than prescribing a bunch of pills. It gave her B complex vitamins, amino acids and trace minerals to treat the cause of her symptoms.

Years later, doctors are still mainly treating symptoms

Even when they suggest better nutrition, it might be based on faulty theories. Doctors think that cholesterol causes heart disease. If a person has high cholesterol, the first thing a doctor says is to stop eating eggs and other healthy foods that contain cholesterol. When that doesn't work, the doctor prescribes a statin drug to keep the liver from making cholesterol.

We need statisticians to correlate the level of "bad" LDL cholesterol with the tremendous increase in sugar consumption, especially high-fructose corn syrup, by the average American. High blood sugar causes high insulin and type II diabetes that produces fatty deposits in arteries all over the body. Isn't it better to remove the true cause of cholesterol and fat deposits - dietary sugars, not fats? With a balanced diet, you will have more energy and fewer disabilities. You can then exercise more and not depend on pills.

If you decide to stay in a big house, consider renting room(s) to another senior citizen or to a college student. One man in his eighties rents a room with kitchen privileges to a student. For a lower-than-market rent, his boarder does a few chores and can call for help in emergencies. If the neighborhood is no longer safe, consider moving to a complex with other seniors. However, there may be decades of papers to go through, as well as rooms full of furniture and other things that you "might use some day." Too bad we no longer have extended families living in big houses, where elders take care of grandchildren and pass along what might be useful, even if it stays in an attic for a generation. Passing along family stories might be even more important. Too many children are getting their values from television instead of from family elders who have gained wisdom from living in a changing world.

Some seniors decide to live in a retirement community. This is expensive, especially if it includes medical care. Few will be able to afford living in a Sun City or similar place that provides both physical and mental stimulation along with companionship.

These activities may well stave off the disabilities of aging.

In the middle 1990s, I visited friends in a large, well-regulated facility near Ashland, Oregon. Residents had the choice of a small house on the grounds or a room in the tower. They had use of the swimming pool, recreation rooms and other facilities. The library included an instrument that changed the printing in a book into sound. Excursions to the Ashland Theatre festival were available, as well as trips to the scenic surroundings. It seemed like a Utopia or an adult summer camp. Maybe it was more like being in a bell jar, untouched by problems of the outside world.

Some seniors find other ways to keep active and involved

A group of older musicians in Roseville, California had made their own instruments to play for nursing home residents. A woman in another community has made books of familiar old songs. An excellent pianist, she plays at sing-a-longs for people in residential facilities.

My friend in Santa Cruz, California, now in her nineties, lives in a manufactured home in a family park. She cultivates flowers but spends most of her time participating in community events. She was one of the founders of the Grey Bears, similar to Senior Gleaners. She has been active in Habitat for Humanity, has taught English to Asian women and is willing and able to participate in demonstrations for better conditions for farm workers. Part of preventing debilitating aging is interacting with others in a meaningful way.

There's more to life than keeping healthy or looking good. Without a purpose exterior to yourself, your life can seem empty and sterile, no matter how pleasant. Why not use the extra vitality from your radiant new health to help others live more fully?

18-3 Ending in a Nursing Home or Other Facility

What happens if your health deteriorates and you can no longer stay in your own home? If you had an adequate income in your working years, you might have bought nursing home insurance. One financial planner says the best time to buy it is in your fifties. Earlier, you're wasting your premiums and after 60 it is too expensive. In 2003, a 40-year-old paid a premium of about $300 a month for this insurance. The nursing care benefit in Medicare is limited to six months following a hospitalization of up to 100 days. As with other federal programs, there are stringent standards for the provider and lots of paper work.

California's Medicaid program is jointly funded by the state and U.S. dollars. It is supposed to be limited to the truly indigent; however, some attorneys say, through radio programs, that you don't have to spend your assets to a poverty level to be eligible. A spouse can remain in the family home and have assets of $70,000. But the state puts a lien on the house and collects after death to make up for what it had spent for the nursing care. This might be greater than the value of the house if the person had a long illness.

Regardless of who pays for it, nursing home life is difficult

It may range from clean and bleak to depressing or even disgusting. In the 1980s, working as a medical technologist for a private laboratory, I was sent to draw blood in several nursing homes. One had beautiful grounds, an impressive entrance, large windows and a spacious sunny reception area. It must have been expensive. However, after the first whiff of incense at the entry, I realized it didn't mask the pervasive smell of urine. Indeed, several of the residents in the television room had urinary bottles fastened to their wheel chairs. Maybe the staff is used to the odor. If this was one of the better homes, imagine what the less expensive ones were like.

When I was a medical student, I visited specific patients in nursing homes. They had been sent there from the county hospital in Denver if they had no acute illness. Before federal standards, most of these nursing homes were big, old houses with only a few rooms and two or three staff members who rotated shifts. The patients were confined to their single or double rooms.

I got to know one old gentleman with a sharp mind who used to read widely. "After my pneumonia, I had to give up my room in the hotel since I couldn't walk up stairs anymore," he told me. "I liked being close to the library and that little café with my friends. I hope there's someplace I can afford when I get out of here."

When I visited him, he was sitting in the dark hallway of the first floor of a Victorian house in an old part of town. What a dismal place it was.

"They have me sit out here when they change the beds," he continued. "The other man in my room is deaf, so I can't even talk to anybody. I sure wish there were enough light to read by. They only turn on the lights at night and they're too dim anyway."

I asked the woman in charge if I could take him for a ride to the park. She refused, saying it was against the rules. I talked with him in the dingy hallway but I left feeling depressed. I visited twice more, then heard he had died of lung cancer. I vowed I would never end up in such a place.

In 1992 I visited one of the nicer facilities in San Diego. My friend was in a single room, about 8 by 10 feet, clean but drab. She didn't recognize me because of her Alzheimer's disease. Her husband said that she was safe and comfortable here, but it cost more than $3,000 a month. Statistics show that Alzheimer's patients can live 10 or more years after diagnosis. It's not much of a life for either spouse. He worried because costs were going up at more than twice the inflation rate. If she had lived to 2003, a month in a nursing home would have cost $6,000. This is more than the retirement pay of many professionals.

During the past 20 years, the concept of Assisted Living Facilities has grown

These are for people who find it difficult to take care of themselves but don't need skilled nursing care. They used to be board and room houses with five or six beds. Now, they can be buildings with several dozen beds that look more like hotels, but feel more inviting. They can take only private patients, but the cost is about half that of a skilled nursing facility. Without the stringent rules of nursing homes, the residents can often have pets.

I saw a video of one such home. Two cats owned by the staff

seemed to brighten the attitude of everyone. Grandchildren were more likely to visit if they could pet the cats. Besides offering room and board, these assisted living facilities can have visiting medical personnel to take care of people recovering from operations or those with chronic medical needs that don't require constant monitoring. Some will take Alzheimer's patients. Security is unobtrusive. Patients wear a monitoring device on wrist or ankle that alerts the staff if they wander to other parts of the building even before they approach an outside door. It's more pleasant to live in a place like this but still expensive.

Don't expect to be saved from a lingering semi-life in a nursing facility either by buying nursing care insurance or by outwitting Medicaid regulations. The nicer places will be expensive and those taking Medicaid may be drab and depressing. Either way, you will have lost your independence as well as your health.

It's up to you to start now to avoid later debilitating illness. Don't think you can smoke, eat fake foods, sweet or starchy manufactured food, fatty meats laced with insecticides or colored drinks loaded with high-fructose corn syrup and expect the pharmaceutical industry to correct what these substances are doing to your body. In addition to eating a healthy diet you must exercise. You can't expect miracle medicines or that medical technology will give you replacement organs. Your body is better than an expensive machine. Nature has developed the body to be healthy if it is given the right nutrients and physical stress. You can't run a Cadillac on whale blubber, so don't try to run your intricate mechanism on junk foods. Do you want to live many years being half-alive?

You can use the following examples for truly golden years:

Penny would be a good role model. She has a zest for life and is active in a local writers' club. She is now writing an article for a magazine about the Mammoth Lakes area in the eastern sierra. She had grown up near there and spent all her summers exploring the natural features. She was impressed with Mammoth Rock and wished to be able to stand on its summit. It was several hundred feet high and the face was a sheer cliff, but she thought there might be a way up on the other side. When she was in her eighties, her son and teen-aged grandsons helped her up a steep rocky trail on the back side. She had achieved her child-hood dream, having fully recovered from hip replacement surgery seven years earlier. The next year they all climbed to Duck Lake, going from 9,000 feet to 10.900 feet. Other hikers struggling up the steep trail were amazed when they heard she was 82.

I have already mentioned Hilda, who is over 90. She rides her bicycle for errands, cooks and does housework and has energy to work for worthy causes.

Ella is in her late nineties and lives in the East Bay. Even though she looks frail, she's not afraid to take Bay Area Rapid Transit trains on Sunday afternoons to attend the San Francisco Opera. She and her late husband always had season tickets and she continues to enjoy one of the world's great opera houses.

Emma, an alert 90-year-old, is neither fat nor frail. She lives in her own home but won't spend any of her late husband's life insurance he said was for her nursing home care. She has had good nutrition for many years. She used to hike and still goes on short walks. She might never need to go to a nursing home, so she could choose to use some of the money to travel or buy something beautiful for her home.

You too can have choices of how you spend your money if you have good health in old age. You won't have to worry if Medicare does or doesn't stay solvent. You have the power to choose the Golden Mean in diet, exercise and lifestyle.

It's up to you: start now to avoid later debilitating illness

The End Result

If you're not yet convinced to forget myths and misinformation and that a quick fix won't last, look at past experiences – yours and others. Don't you want to lead a vital energetic life as long as you're here? The future is yours to modify by changing your ideas and behavior.

An unrealistic body ideal has made healthy people of normal weight want to be thin. They cut their calories and some start smoking. They become too thin, anorexic or bulimic. With lower metabolism, they fight fat the rest of their lives. Then they become obese and develop metabolic problems such as diabetes, cardiovascular disease and cancer.

Excessive exercise to get thin is also harmful. Too much running can deplete the immune system and cause colds. It can lead to decreased bone density with fractures. It decreases normal body fat and causes hormone imbalances, especially in women so they stop menstruating.

Carbohydrate foods form glucose. With too much glucose, insulin rises too high and eventually, all body cells become resistant to insulin. Excess insulin is then produced. This damages blood vessels. Meanwhile, the liver changes the excess glucose to body fat. Cholesterol is deposited to repair the damage in blood vessel walls. High-fructose corn syrup is even more damaging. The liver easily makes it into fat and the "bad" low-density cholesterol.

Faulty diets with too many processed foods are especially dangerous

These contain trans fats, either hydrogenated or partially hydrogenated, along with too many starches and sugars. These trans fats can replace the natural fats in the cells of your artery walls and make them less elastic and more prone to developing tears that cause blood clots to adhere. LDL cholesterol then collects and causes cardiovascular disease. Natural saturated fats like butter and coconut oil along with essential omega-3 and omega-6 fatty acids from oils help make normal cell membranes that resist injury.

The low-saturated fat, high-carbohydrate diet of the past 30 years has resulted in more obesity, more diabetes and more heart disease. You don't have to continue down that path.

The very low-carbohydrate, high-protein Atkins diet is another extreme diet with different dangers. It is being used by millions to lose weight. It is not a magic way to lose fat without exercising. Muscle burns fat at rest but much more during exercise. The large amount of meat puts high levels of fixed acids from nitrates and phosphates into your blood. This can cause calcium to come out of your bones to counterbalance these mineral acids.

Taking calcium pills won't help unless you exercise. They might not be absorbed to be deposited into your bones to replace daily calcium loss. Phosphates in diet soft drinks will also remove calcium from your bones. As you lose weight on a high-protein diet, you might look better with less body fat but get osteoporosis and be more prone to hip fractures. As millions try the Atkins diet, they might have early weight loss, but will later suffer adverse effects of this extreme approach to eating. They are already making their livers and kidneys work harder to rid the body of the urea and uric acid from excess proteins. Unless they avoid meat from factory farms, they will get an overdose of insecticides and antibiotics dissolved in the animals' fat.

Costs of surgical procedures and prescription pills keep increasing much faster than the general cost of living

Metabolic diseases could have been prevented with a better, more natural diet, more exercise and a lifestyle that reduces stress.

It's time for you to look at your lifestyle and take charge of your own health. Then you won't be dependent on a medical system that leaves one-fifth of Americans without health insurance and charges everyone else higher premiums. It's time for you to practice prevention. As the number of retired persons doubles, the U.S. won't be able to afford expensive heart surgery, organ transplants or many prescriptions that cost several hundred dollars per person per month.

Heart disease has increased despite diets low in saturated fat and cholesterol.

The great reduction of smoking in men during the past 40 years should have cut down on heart disease as well as lung cancer. Women though are smoking more (to get thin) and both are suffering from more heart disease. Lung cancer is a leading cancer in women and harder to treat than breast cancer.

The following anecdote might help you make up your mind:

I heard a talk by a motivator of real estate sales people in the 1980s. He asked us to suppose that a good friend told you he had to be out of town for several weeks and you're the only one he trusts with his pure-bred dog. He continued: Would you keep the dog in a smoky room, give him heavily sugared black coffee or colas, candy bars and potato chips during the day and a highball at night? Of course not! You would feed the dog only the well-balanced food the owner provided. Would you put the dog in a small space where all he could do was stand, sit or lie down? Of course not! You would exercise the dog.

Why then do you treat your own body in the wrong way, subsisting on stimulants, junk foods and maybe a few vitamin pills? Your health is just as important as that of a dog. No amount of income can replace good health. Of course you should devote your weekends to your clients, but you should schedule time during the week for yourself and activities with your family. Gaining and keeping good health helps your selling ability in the long-term and gives you a balanced life.

I thought of two successful women real estate brokers. One,

in her late fifties had a nice office and concentrated on selling homes in an upscale San Diego suburb. She drove an expensive car, lived in a large house, wore lots of gold jewelry and seemed the epitome of success. Later, as a smoker with a puffy, overweight body, she died in her sixties. What good were those external trappings of success?

The other woman was under forty. She chose to sell commercial properties, leaving weekends free. She and a man friend bought a boat and joined two water-ski clubs. She got plenty of exercise in the fresh air and made contacts with builders and investors who also enjoyed the sport. I predict she will keep her good figure and easily weather the ups and downs of a stressful profession. Exercise and healthy living do work.

Keep in mind the following thoughts to help change your ideas and activities:

- Dieting produces obesity. Low-calorie diets slow down your metabolism and cause you to lose muscle first and fat later.

- Beware of the "easy" calories in sweet drinks, desserts, deep-fried foods and alcohol.

- Eat natural foods. Cut way back or eliminate manufactured foods.

- Eat plenty of vegetables, but lesser amounts of fruit and high-fiber, whole-grain foods.

- Eat a protein food (meat, eggs, cheese, tofu, beans, seeds or nuts) with every meal or snack. Daily meat or fish portions should be no bigger than the size of your palm.

- Eat whole foods, not juices, for their fiber and more antioxidants as well as vitamins and minerals.

- Use milkshake diet drinks only in emergency. They have no fiber or fat and too many sugars.

- Get 30 percent of your calories from fat. Eat essential omega-3 fatty acids in flax or flax oil, fatty fish or walnuts. Use olive oil, canola oil, peanut oil or butter. Avoid most poly-unsaturated vegetable oils and the trans fats made from them.

- Move your body more. Try for 10,000 steps a day. Drive less. Use the stairs.

- Try a strength building exercise twice a week. Use weights or work against gravity or do yard work manually without machines.

- Combine aerobic and strength building exercise by hiking or bicycling uphill.

- Do yoga or other flexibility exercise to move each joint through its complete range.

- Maintain balance and coordination by dancing or playing your favorite sport.

- Avoid environmental toxins. Be wary of household products with scent or shine.

- Take 5 to 20 minutes a day to close your eyes and meditate or just take long slow breaths.

- Try to see every interaction from another person's point of view.

- Laugh or at least try to smile. It can relieve stress.

- Do something for someone else. Express love to people or pets.

- Change your value system. Doing things with your family or others is more important than having more possessions.

- Have both long-term and short-term goals for the remainder of your life.

Consider the following alternatives:

- Which do you want, the short-term pleasure of sweet drinks and daily desserts or long-term freedom from medication for diabetes and other metabolic diseases?

- Would you rather spend your time walking and doing other exercise or sit watching other people on television? A passive life is half a life.

- Would you like to spend your retirement years enjoying activities with other people or sitting alone, restricted by your pill-taking schedule or your numerous ailments?

Your greatest power is the POWER TO CHOOSE

The results of your choices may take a long time to show up but they will appear.

Your body is meant to be healthy if you give it a chance.

You don't need to be a rigid ascetic to avoid being overly self-indulgent. Enjoy forbidden foods once a month or on special occasions and really appreciate them.

Live a full healthy life by avoiding extremes.

Aim for the Golden Mean

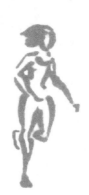

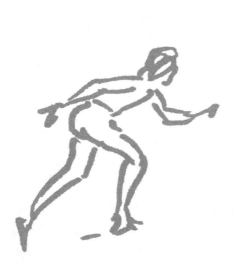

Oldways Preservation Trust
4 Food Pyramids

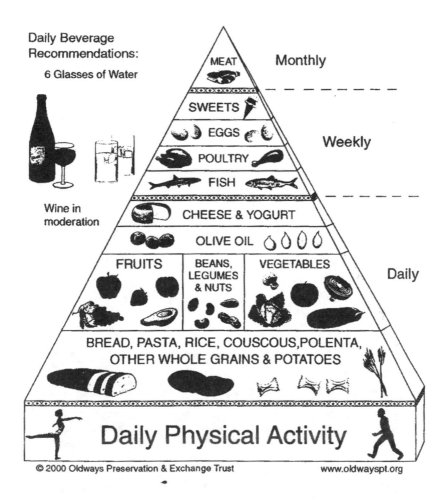

The Traditional Healthy Mediterranean Diet Pyramid

Daily Beverage Recommendations:

6 Glasses of Water

Wine in moderation

MEAT — Monthly

SWEETS

EGGS
POULTRY
FISH — Weekly

CHEESE & YOGURT

OLIVE OIL

FRUITS | BEANS, LEGUMES & NUTS | VEGETABLES — Daily

BREAD, PASTA, RICE, COUSCOUS, POLENTA, OTHER WHOLE GRAINS & POTATOES

Daily Physical Activity

© 2000 Oldways Preservation & Exchange Trust   www.oldwayspt.org

The Traditional Healthy
Latin American Diet Pyramid

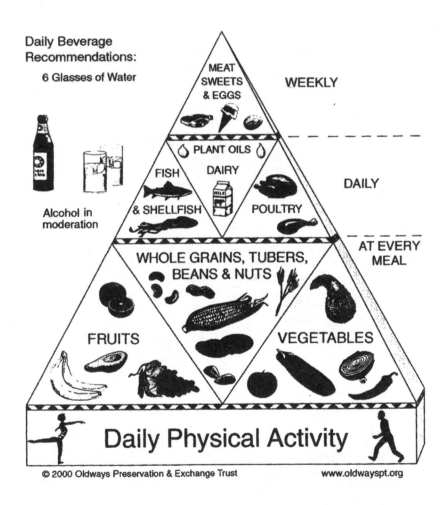

Daily Beverage
Recommendations:

6 Glasses of Water

Alcohol in
moderation

MEAT
SWEETS
& EGGS

WEEKLY

PLANT OILS

DAIRY

FISH
& SHELLFISH

POULTRY

DAILY

WHOLE GRAINS, TUBERS,
BEANS & NUTS

AT EVERY
MEAL

FRUITS

VEGETABLES

Daily Physical Activity

© 2000 Oldways Preservation & Exchange Trust   www.oldwayspt.org

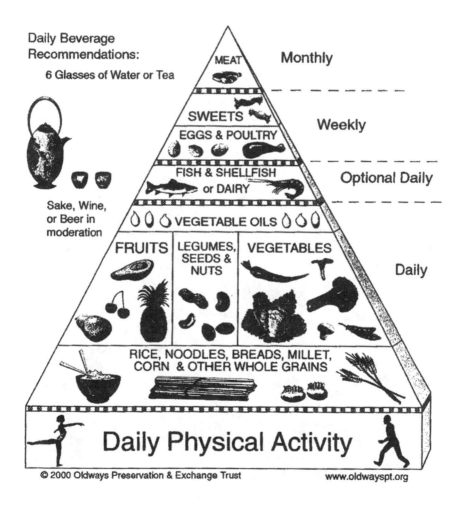

The Traditional Healthy Asian Diet Pyramid

Daily Beverage Recommendations:

6 Glasses of Water or Tea

Sake, Wine, or Beer in moderation

MEAT — Monthly

SWEETS

EGGS & POULTRY — Weekly

FISH & SHELLFISH or DAIRY — Optional Daily

VEGETABLE OILS

FRUITS | LEGUMES, SEEDS & NUTS | VEGETABLES — Daily

RICE, NOODLES, BREADS, MILLET, CORN & OTHER WHOLE GRAINS

Daily Physical Activity

© 2000 Oldways Preservation & Exchange Trust   www.oldwayspt.org

The Traditional Healthy
Vegetarian Diet Pyramid

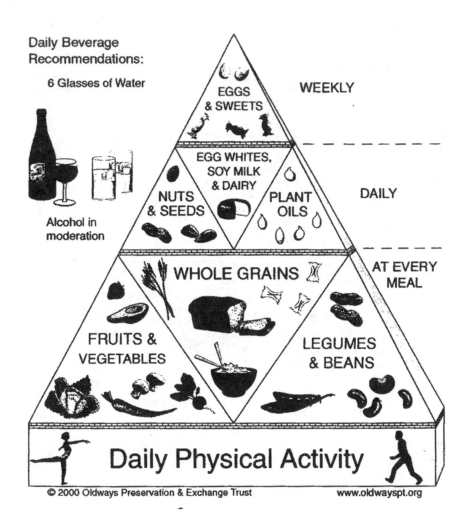

Daily Beverage
Recommendations:

6 Glasses of Water

Alcohol in
moderation

WEEKLY

EGGS
& SWEETS

EGG WHITES,
SOY MILK
& DAIRY

NUTS
& SEEDS

PLANT
OILS

DAILY

WHOLE GRAINS

AT EVERY
MEAL

FRUITS &
VEGETABLES

LEGUMES
& BEANS

Daily Physical Activity

© 2000 Oldways Preservation & Exchange Trust   www.oldayspt.org

Janeen Hunt's Annotated Bibliography on Fat & Cholesterol

A Review of Diet, Fat, and Cholesterol Research: Twenty-Five Points

Introduction:

Those who have heart disease generally but not always have high blood cholesterol. It is therefore theorized that high cholesterol causes heart disease. This is called a correlation. One type of correlation is an observation where when something increases, something else increases (a positive association) or when something increases, something else decreases (an inverse association).

An example of how correlations don't necessarily prove anything is: In the last 100 years there has been an increase in global warming. And in the last 100 years women's shoe sizes have gotten bigger.

Does this show that global warming causes women's feet to get bigger?

So does high cholesterol cause heart disease? Just because many people have high cholesterol that also have heart disease doesn't prove this. Heart disease could cause high cholesterol. Or else high cholesterol could be a normal state for some people and heart disease could be caused by some other factor that causes cholesterol to clog the arteries. This is not a speculative statement as there exist at least two theories of heart disease that may make cholesterol an insignificant factor in heart disease: the homocysteine theory and the C-reactive protein theory.[1, 2, 8, 3]

1. Total serum cholesterol has proven not to be a strong determinant of cardiovascular risk.[4, 5]

2. HDL ratio has been proven to be a better standard to assess cardiovascular risk.[6] What can you eat to raise HDL? Only one thing: fat.[7] All fats raise HDL but saturated fats raise HDL the most.[6]

3. The saturated fats except stearic acid do raise total serum cholesterol levels as shown in controlled and epidemiological studies.[8, 9, 10, 23, 39] This is insignificant if total cholesterol has little to do with heart disease.

4. If you have high cholesterol in most cases there is no need to avoid red meat. This is because only 30% of fats in red meat are composed of the saturated fats that raise cholesterol. What are the other 70%? Stearic acid which has a neutral effect on cholesterol comprises about 15%.[8, 23] About 50% is monounsaturated fat (like olive oil) which does not raise total cholesterol levels but raises HDL the good cholesterol.[31] And the remainder is polyunsaturated fat which lowers total cholesterol levels while raising HDL.[11] One study shows that lean red meat is equal to eating lean white meat.[12] So how do they test whether saturated fats raise cholesterol if red meat has so much of the other fats? One study used tropical oils.[10] Others have used liquid cholesterol products. When a natural diet is used, calculations are made according to percentage of each fat in each product, then elevation of cholesterol is apportioned accordingly.

5. It is beneficial that some saturated fats can raise cholesterol because if blood cholesterol gets too low, people get depressed, commit suicide or die from cancer or stroke.[13, 14, 15, 16]

6. Studies are inconsistent regarding saturated fat.[4] In one epidemiological study the more saturated fat one ate, the lower their serum cholesterol was.[17] In another study, saturated fats in the diet were high, but serum cholesterol levels were low.[18] Because the results of studies are lacking consistency as regards to saturated fats in the diet, there must be some attenuating

affect of saturated fats that negates the rise in total serum cholesterol.[23, 22]

7. It is over-simplifying to name one villain, "saturated fat", as the culprit in heart disease especially when the results of studies on saturated fat are contradictory, inconclusive, and ambiguous at best.[19, 20, 21] There are other factors that influence heart disease including but not limited to high glycemic carbohydrate intake, homocysteine, C-reactive protein, oxidative stress, smoking, and exercise to name just a few.[51] A meta-analysis of research to date states, "Despite decades of effort and many thousands of people randomized, there is still only limited and inconclusive evidence of the effects of modification of total, saturated, monounsaturated, or polyunsaturated fats on cardiovascular morbidity and mortality."[5]

8. In most people, however, if saturated fat raises their blood cholesterol it is probably not an important risk factor for heart disease as HDL is raised along with total cholesterol. It is also important to note that although LDL is raised too, it has been shown that there are two different types of LDL and saturated fats raise the good kind of LDL.[22] Also avoiding saturated fat may not be an important deterrent to heart disease because saturated fat is never isolated in natural animal products but accompanied by monounsaturated (olive-oil-type) fats. Therefore, the combination of fats in animal products keep cholesterol levels where they should be which accounts for them not being a significant risk factor.[23]

9. Fat intake in the diet should not be decreased.[24, 23, 25, 49, 26] Lowering saturated fats and cholesterol in the diet lowers HDL and decreases secretion of the good APO A-1 cholesterol.[27, 28]

10. Protein with 80% from animal products which includes saturated fats lessens risk of heart disease.[29, 30]

11. Replacing saturated fats in the diet with carbohydrates is bad for your serum cholesterol and bad in general for your heart disease risk and mortality.[31, 32, 33, 34, 35, 36, 49] Carbohydrates are not an essential nutrient in the diet.[37] Carbohydrates increase C-reactive protein thereby increasing risk of heart disease.[38]

12. Some nations that eat a high amount of fats and animal products (Crete[39, 40, 4] and Spain[41]) have less heart disease than nations who eat a little fat. Total fat in the diet is not an indicator.[4, 24]

13. Dietary cholesterol has little impact on total blood cholesterol.[42] Dietary cholesterol does not increase risk for heart disease or stroke.[43] Two-thirds of the population show no change in serum cholesterol levels from intake of cholesterol.[44] Dietary cholesterol accounts for a minimum amount of cholesterol produced by the body. The liver produces most cholesterol in the body. Eating cholesterol down-regulates your body's production of cholesterol.[45]

14. Many people with low cholesterol levels die of heart disease. One article stated: "Indeed, high cholesterol levels alone could only predict at most half of all heart attacks."[2] Many people with exceptionally elevated levels of cholesterol never have a heart attack.[2]

15. Researchers say if a person, group of people or nation has higher serum cholesterol that they are at greater risk for heart disease. Croatia and Japan have high cholesterol but low heart disease.[46, 47] But considering that many people have high cholesterol and do not have heart disease and many with low cholesterol do have heart disease, then this may not be a valid marker of risk.[2]

16. Once the rise in HDL is factored in, studies have shown that saturated fats are less of a risk factor for heart disease than carbohydrate.[23, 48, 49]

17. Many people with heart disease have high triglycerides. High triglycerides are a risk factor for heart disease.[50, 51, 52] Eating fat, any kind of fat, lowers triglycerides.[23, 53]

18. There is one fat that should be avoided: trans fat (partially hydrogenated oil). Replacement of just 2% of energy from trans unsaturated fats with unsaturated fats would result in a 53% risk reduction for coronary heart disease.[25] The U.S. government Board of Food and Nutrition recently issued a report on trans fat saying "that dietary trans fatty acids are more deleterious with

respect to coronary heart disease than saturated fatty acids."[54] This report suggests "a Tolerable Upper Intake Level (UL) of zero."[55]

19. Although the government's Dietary Guidelines for Americans recommends that Americans cut their daily saturated fat intake to 10% and certain researchers recommend replacing saturated fat with polyunsaturated fat, there appear to be valid reasons to fear replacing saturated fats with polyunsaturated fats.[56, 49] When the arterial plaque of deceased humans was examined it contained polyunsaturated fats.[57] Oxidation of fats whether it occurs in the body or whether oxidized fat is ingested is known to lead to clogging of the arteries. The fat that oxidizes the easiest is polyunsaturated fat.[58] Saturated fats are the most stable.[59]

20. The American Heart Association has recommended that people with low HDL go on a diet high in unsaturated fat rather than replacing fat with carbohydrate.[60]

21. Saturated fats do not increase risk of diabetes.[61] The American Diabetes Association has recently recommended a high monounsaturated fat diet to those with diabetes.[62]

22. The American Heart Association says high glycemic carbohydrates are linked to heart disease.[63]

23. The American Heart Association says Americans should eat a 30% fat diet with not less than 15% fat.[60] The American Heart Association says diets less than 15% fat can be dangerous.[64] Ironically, Americans do not know this so they try to eat 0% fat and are ruining their health. However, these guidelines limiting fat intake to 30% do not appear to have support of the studies shown here.

24. Fats are not the cause of obesity.[65, 66] Studies have shown that diets high in fat and low in carbohydrate cause a person to lose weight.[67] High fat foods like nuts decrease risk of heart disease.[68]

25. Another important consideration is what our bodies were meant to eat. For the last 2.5 million years man has evolved as a hunter/gatherer with emphasis on carnivore-hunter. In the past hundred years man may have evolved a higher conscious-

ness and may want to be vegetarian, but our bodies are genetically still 99.8% Paleolithic man and as such require meat. The leading experts on Paleolithic Nutrition say that man has eaten mostly animal products (likely over 50%) for most of his existence on earth.[69, 70, 71] Another important factor in evolution was man's development of a larger brain vs. body size. The only way this could have happened was with a nutrient dense source. The accepted explanation is "The Expensive Tissue Hypothesis" which states that meat and fat were that source.[72] These studies show that during man's entire history on earth fat intake would have exceeded both carbohydrate and protein intake. Grains are a foreign product in human evolution. For 99.9% of man's existence on earth, man did not eat grain. In fact, man is the only primate to eat cereal grains.[73] Therefore, trying to force our bodies to accept some form of higher consciousness by trying not to eat animal products would be a foreign diet to our system causing an unbalance and malnutrition in ways that science cannot even predict. Imbalance in the human body is the cause of all disease. When the body is perfectly balanced it is disease-free. Imbalance causes cancer, heart disease, autoimmune disease, and death. In other words, man's so-called recent "higher consciousness" is killing him.

Therefore, fat in the diet has never been the problem. Avoiding fat is the problem.

References

[1] McCully KS, Wilson RB. *Homocysteine theory of arteriosclerosis,* Atherosclerosis 1975 Sep-Oct;22(2):215-27.

[2] Gary Taubes, *Does Inflammation Cut to the Heart of the Matter?* Science Magazine Volume 296, Number 5566, Issue of 12 Apr 2002, pp. 242-245.

[3] Rost NS, Wolf PA, Kase CS, Kelly-Hayes M, Silbershatz H, Massaro JM, D'Agostino RB, Franzblau C, Wilson PW. *Plasma concentration of C-reactive protein and risk of ischemic stroke and transient ischemic attack: the Framingham study.* Stroke 2001 Nov;32(11):2575-9.

[4] Hu FB, Manson JE, Willett WC, *Types of dietary fat and risk of coronary heart disease: a critical review.* J Am Coll Nutr 2001 Feb;20(1):5-19.

[5] Lee Hooper et al, *Dietary fat intake and prevention of cardiovascular disease: systematic review.* BMJ 2001;322:757-763 (31 March).

[6] Ridker PM, Stampfer MJ, Rifai N. *Novel risk factors for systemic atherosclerosis: a comparison of C-reactive protein, fibrinogen, homocysteine, lipoprotein(a), and standard cholesterol screening as predictors of peripheral arterial disease*. JAMA 2001 May 16;285(19):2481-5.

[7] Niacin also raises HDL. Tavvintharan S, Kashyap ML, *The benefits of niacin in atherosclerosis*. Curr Atheroscler Rep 2001 Jan; 3(1):74-82.

[8] Pai T, Yeh YY, *Stearic acid unlike shorter-chain saturated fatty acids is poorly utilized for triacylglycerol synthesis and beta-oxidation in cultured rat hepatocytes*. Lipids 1996 Feb;31(2):159-64.

[9] Kelly FD, Sinclair AJ, Mann NJ, Turner AH, Raffin FL, Blandford MV, Pike MJ. *Short-term diets enriched in stearic or palmitic acids do not alter plasma lipids, platelet aggregation or platelet activation status.* Eur J Clin Nutr 2002 Jun;56(6):490-9.

[10] Francisco J. Sánchez-Muniz, Mari Cruz Merinero, Sonia Rodríguez-Gil, Jose M Ordovas, Sofía Ródenas and Carmen Cuesta, *Dietary Fat Saturation Affects Apolipoprotein AII Levels and HDL Composition in Postmenopausal Women.* The American Society for Nutritional Sciences. J. Nutr. 132:50-54, 2002.

[11] Gary Taubes, *The Soft Science of Dietary Fat Science.* Volume 291, Number 5513, Issue of 30 Mar 2001, pp. 2536-2545.

[12] Davidson MH, Hunninghake D, Maki KC, Kwiterovich PO Jr, Kafonek S, *Comparison of the effects of lean red meat vs lean white meat on serum lipid levels among free-living persons with hypercholesterolemia: a long-term, randomized clinical trial.* Arch Intern Med 1999 Jun 28;159(12):1331-8..

[13] Kreger BE, Anderson KM, Schatzkin A, Splansky GL.Cancer, *Serum cholesterol level, body mass index, and the risk of colon cancer. The Framingham Study.* 1992 Sep 1;70(5):1038-43

[14] Hawthon K, Cowen P, Owens D, Bond A, Elliott M. *Low serum cholesterol and suicide.* Br J Psychiatry 1993 Jun;162:818-25.

[15] Ellison LF, Morrison HI, *Low serum cholesterol concentration and risk of suicide.* Epidemiology 2001 Mar;12(2):168-72.

[16] Iso H, Stampfer MJ, Manson JE, Rexrode K, Hu F, Hennekens CH, Colditz GA, Speizer FE, Willett WC. *Prospective study of fat and protein intake and risk of intraparenchymal hemorrhage in women.* Circulation 2001 Feb 13;103(6):856-63.

[17] Castelli, William, *Concerning the Possibility of a Nut...,* Archives of Internal Med, Jul 1992, 152:(7):1371-2.

[18] Posner BM, Cupples LA, Franz MM, Gagnon DR. *Diet and heart disease risk factors in adult American men and women: the Framingham Offspring-Spouse nutrition studies*. Int J Epidemiol 1993 Dec;22(6):1014-25.

[19] Pietinen P, Ascherio A, Korhonen P, Hartman AM, Willett WC, Albanes D, Vir-

tamo J. *Intake of fatty acids and risk of coronary heart disease in a cohort of Finnish men*. The Alpha-Tocopherol, Beta-Carotene Cancer Prevention Study. Am J Epidemiol 1997 May 15;145(10):876-87.

[20] Ascherio A, Rimm EB, Giovannucci EL, Spiegelman D, Stampfer M, Willett WC. *Dietary fat and risk of coronary heart disease in men: cohort follow up study in the United States*. BMJ 1996 Jul 13;313(7049):84-90.

[21] Fehily AM, Yarnell JW, Sweetnam PM, Elwood PC. *Diet and incident isch-aemic heart disease: the Caerphilly Study*. Br J Nutr 1993 Mar;69(2):303-14.

[22] Dreon DM, Fernstrom HA, Campos H, Blanche P, Williams PT, Krauss RM. *Change in dietary saturated fat intake is correlated with change in mass of large low-density-lipoprotein particles in men*. Am J Clin Nutr 1998 May;67(5):828-36.

[23] Mensink et al. *Effect of dietary fatty acids on serum lipids and lipoproteins. A meta-analysis of 27 trials*. Arterioscler Thromb 1992; 12: 911-9. Quote from conclusion: "Surprisingly, our regression equation would predict that replacement of saturates by carbohydrates yields little if any improvement in coronary risk."

[24] L.A. Corr, M.F. Oliver, *The low fat/low cholesterol diet is ineffective*, European Heart Journal European Heart Journal (1997) 18, 18-22.

[25] Hu FB, Stampfer MJ, Manson JE, Rimm E, Colditz GA, Rosner BA, Hennekens CH, Willett WC. *Dietary fat intake and the risk of coronary heart disease in women*. N Engl J Med 1997 Nov 20;337(21):1491-9.

[26] Gillman MW, Cupples LA, Millen BE, Ellison RC, Wolf PA. *Inverse association of dietary fat with development of ischemic stroke in men*. JAMA 1997 Dec 24-31;278(24):2145-50.

[27] Velez-Carrasco W, Lichtenstein AH, Welty FK, Li Z, Lamon-Fava S, Dolnikowski GG, Schaefer EJ. *Dietary restriction of saturated fat and cholesterol decreases HDL ApoA-I secretion.* Arterioscler Thromb Vasc Biol 1999 Apr;19(4):918-24.

[28] Brinton E, S. E., Jan Breslow (1990). *A Low-fat Diet Decreases High Density Lipoprotein (HDL) Cholesterol Levels by Decreasing HDL Apolipoprotein Transport Rates*. J Clin. Invest. 85(January): 144-151.

[29] Frank B Hu, Meir J Stampfer, JoAnn E Manson, Eric Rimm, Graham A Colditz, Frank E Speizer, Charles H Hennekens and Walter C Willett. *Dietary protein and risk of ischemic heart disease in women.* American Journal of Clinical Nutrition, Vol. 70, No. 2, 221-227, August 1999.

[30] Frank B Hu and Walter Willett. *Reply to TC Campbell*. American Journal of Clinical Nutrition, Vol. 71, No. 3, 850-851, March 2000.

[31] Kris-Etherton PM. *AHA Science Advisory: monounsaturated fatty acids and risk of cardiovascular disease.* American Heart Association Nutrition Committee. *Circulation..* 1999;100:1253–1258

[32] Simin Liu, JoAnn E Manson, Frank B Hu and Walter C Willett. *Reply to DL Katz*. American Journal of Clinical Nutrition, Vol. 73, No. 1, 132-133, January 2001.

[33] Liu S, Willett WC, Stampfer MJ, et al. *A prospective study of dietary glycemic load, carbohydrate intake, and risk of coronary heart disease in US women*. Am J Clin Nutr 2000,71:1455–61.

[34] Simin Liu, JoAnn E Manson, Frank B Hu and Walter C Willett, *Reply to BO Schneeman*, American Journal of Clinical Nutrition, Vol. 73, No. 1, 130-131, January 2001.

[35] J Jeppesen, P Schaaf, C Jones, MY Zhou, YD Chen and GM Reaven, *Effects of low-fat, high-carbohydrate diets on risk factors for ischemic heart disease in postmenopausal women.* American Journal of Clinical Nutrition, Vol 65, 1027-1033, 1997.

[36] MB Katan, *Effect of low-fat diets on plasma high-density lipoprotein concentrations*. American Journal of Clinical Nutrition, Vol 67, 573S-576S, 1998.

[37] Eric C Westman, *Is dietary carbohydrate essential for human nutrition?* American Journal of Clinical Nutrition, Vol. 75, No. 5, 951-953, May 2002.

[38] Simin Liu, JoAnn E Manson, Julie E Buring, Meir J Stampfer, Walter C Willett and Paul M Ridker, *Relation between a diet with a high glycemic load and plasma concentrations of high-sensitivity C-reactive protein in middle-aged women.* American Journal of Clinical Nutrition, Vol. 75, No. 3, 492-498, March 2002.

[39] Keys A, *Seven Countries: A Multivariate Analysis of Death and Coronary Heart Disease*, Cambridge, MA, Haarvard University Press, 1980.

[40] Kafatos A, Diacatou A, Voukiklaris G, Nikolakakis N, Vlachonikolis J, Kounali D, Mamalakis G, Dontas AS. *Heart disease risk-factor status and dietary changes in the Cretan population over the past 30 y: the Seven Countries Study*. Am J Clin Nutr 1997 Jun;65(6):1882-6.

[41] L Serra-Majem, L Ribas, R Tresserras, J Ngo and L Salleras. *How could changes in diet explain changes in coronary heart disease mortality in Spain? The Spanish paradox.* American Journal of Clinical Nutrition, Vol 61, 1351S-1359S, 1995.

[42] Boucher P, de Lorgeril M, Salen P, Crozier P, Delaye J, Vallon JJ, Geyssant A, Dante R.
Effect of dietary cholesterol on low density lipoprotein-receptor, 3-hydroxy-3-methylglutaryl-CoA reductase, and low density lipoprotein receptor-related protein mRNA expression in healthy humans. Lipids 1998 Dec;33(12):1177-86.

[43] Hu FB, Stampfer MJ, Rimm EB, Manson JE, Ascherio A, Colditz GA, Rosner BA, Spiegelman D, Speizer FE, Sacks FM, Hennekens CH, Willett WC. *A prospective study of egg consumption and risk of cardiovascular disease in men*

and women. JAMA 1999 Apr 21;281(15):1387-94.

[44] McNamara DJ. *Dietary cholesterol and the optimal diet for reducing risk of atherosclerosis.* Can J Cardiol 1995 Oct;11 Suppl G:123G-126G.

[45] Jones PJ, Pappu AS, Hatcher L, Li ZC, Illingworth DR, Connor WE, *Dietary cholesterol feeding suppresses human cholesterol synthesis measured by deuterium incorporation and urinary mevalonic acid levels.* Arterioscler Thromb Vasc Biol 1996 Oct;16(10):1222-8.

[46] Menotti A, Keys A, Blackburn H, Kromhout D, Karvonen M, Nissinen A, Pekkanen J, Punsar S, Fidanza F, Giampaoli S, Seccareccia F, Buzina R, Mohacek I, Nedeljkovic S, Aravanis C, Dontas A, Toshima H, Lanti M. *Comparison of multivariate predictive power of major risk factors for coronary heart diseases in different countries: results from eight nations of the Seven Countries Study, 25-year follow-up.* J Cardiovasc Risk 1996 Feb;3(1):69-75.

[47] Verschuren WM, Jacobs DR, Bloemberg BP, Kromhout D, Menotti A, Aravanis C, Blackburn H, Buzina R, Dontas AS, Fidanza F, et al. *Serum total cholesterol and long-term coronary heart disease mortality in different cultures. Twenty-five-year follow-up of the seven countries study.* JAMA 1995 Jul 12;274(2):131-6.

[48] Walter C Willett, *Reply to AE Hardman.* American Journal of Clinical Nutrition, Vol. 72, No. 4, 1061-1062, October 2000.

[49] Walter C. Willett, *Will High-Carbohydrate/Low-Fat Diets Reduce the Risk of Coronary Heart Disease?* Proc Soc Exp Biol Med 2000 Dec; 225(3):187-90.

[50] Lapidus L, Bengtsson C, Lindquist O, Sigurdsson JA, Rybo E. *Triglycerides--main lipid risk factor for cardiovascular disease in women?* Acta Med Scand 1985;217(5):481-9.

[51] Harjai KJ. *Potential new cardiovascular risk factors : left ventricular hypertrophy, homocysteine, lipoprotein(a), triglycerides , oxidative stress, and fibrinogen.* Ann Intern Med 1999 Sep 7;131(5):376-86.

[52] Cullen P., *Evidence that triglycerides are an independent coronary heart disease risk factor.* Am J Cardiol 2000 Nov 1;86(9):943-9.

[53] Walter Willett, Meir Stampfer, Nain-Feng Chu, Donna Spiegelman, Michelle Holmes and Eric Rimm, *Assessment of Questionnaire Validity for Measuring Total Fat Intake using Plasma Lipid Levels as Criteria.* American Journal of Epidemiology Vol. 154, No. 12 : 1107-1112, 2001.

[54] Ascherio A, Hennekens CH, Buring JE, Master C, Stampfer MJ, Willett WC. 1994. *Trans fatty acids intake and risk of myocardial infarction.* Circulation 89:94–101.

[55] Letter Report on Dietary Reference Intakes for *Trans* Fatty Acids; Institute of Medicine in the National Academy of Sciences, July 10, 2002. http://www.iom.edu/iom/iomhome.nsf/Pages/FNB+Reports.

[56] *Dietary Guidelines for Americans* http://www.nal.usda.gov/fnic/dga/dga95/lowfat.html

[57] Felton CV et al: Dietary polyunsaturated fatty acids and composition of human aortic plaques. Lancet 1994; 344:1195-1196.

[58] Nippon Rinsho, *Modified low-density lipoprotein*. 1994 Dec; 52(12):3090-5.

[59] Bourre JM, Piciotti M. *Alterations in eighteen-carbon saturated, mono-unsaturated and polyunsaturated fatty acid peroxisomal oxidation in mouse brain during development and aging.* Biochem Mol Biol Int 1997 Mar;41(3):461-8.

[60] Ronald M. Krauss, et al, *AHA Dietary Guidelines : Revision 2000: A Statement for Healthcare Professionals From the Nutrition Committee of the American Heart Association* Circulation 0: 2296-2311.

[61] Salmeron J, Hu FB, Manson JE, Stampfer MJ, Colditz GA, Rimm EB, Willett WC. *Dietary fat intake and risk of type 2 diabetes in women*. Am J Clin Nutr 2001 Jun;73(6):1019-26.

[62] Marion J. Franz, et al. *Evidence-Based Nutrition Principles and Recommendations for the Treatment and Prevention of Diabetes and Related Complications* Diabetes Care 25:148-198, 2002.

[63] Barbara V. Howard, PhD; Judith Wylie-Rosett, RD, EdD *AHA Scientific Statement Sugar and Cardiovascular Disease A Statement for Healthcare Professionals From the Committee on Nutrition of the Council on Nutrition, Physical Activity, and Metabolism of the American Heart Association* Circulation. 2002;106:523

[64] *Very low fat diets may harm some people*. BMJ 1998 Feb 21;316(7131):573

[65] Willett WC *Dietary fat plays a major role in obesity: No.* Obesity Review 2002 May;3(2):59-68.

[66] Walter C Willett *Is dietary fat a major determinant of body fat?* Am J Clin Nutr 1998;67(suppl):556S–62S. 1998

[67] Westman EC, Yancy WS, Edman JS, Tomlin KF, Perkins CE, *Effect of 6-month adherence to a very low carbohydrate diet program*. Am J Med 2002 Jul;113(1):30-6.

[68] Hu FB, Stampfer MJ, Manson JE, Rimm EB, Colditz GA, Rosner BA, Speizer FE, Hennekens CH, Willett WC. *Frequent nut consumption and risk of coronary heart disease in women: prospective cohort study*. BMJ 1998 Nov 14;317(7169):1341-5.

[69] Loren Cordain, Janette Brand Miller, S Boyd Eaton, Neil Mann, Susanne HA Holt and John D Speth *Plant-animal subsistence ratios and macronutrient energy estimations in worldwide hunter-gatherer diets.* American Journal of Clinical Nutrition, Vol. 71, No. 3, 682-692, March 2000.

[70] Cordain L, Eaton SB, Miller JB, Mann N, Hill K. *The paradoxical nature of hunter-gatherer diets: meat-based, yet non-atherogenic.* Eur J Clin Nutr

2002 Mar;56 Suppl 1:S42-52.

[71] Loren Cordain, Janette Brand Miller, S Boyd Eaton and Neil Mann *Macronutrient estimations in hunter-gatherer diets* American Journal of Clinical Nutrition, Vol. 72, No. 6, 1589-1590, December 2000.

[72] Aiello LC, Wheeler PE. *The expensive-tissue hypothesis.* Current Anthropol 36:199-221, 1995.

[73] S. Boyd Eaton, MD, Stanley B. Eaton III *Evolution, Diet and Health* , poster session, the Williamsburg-ICAES conference 1998.

Personal Food Choices & Suggestions

Most health books have many pages of suggested menus and recipes. Some people like to be told what to eat and when. They are already too fixated on food. They shop using a carbohydrate counter as well as a list of total calories in a variety of foods. They weigh or measure foods at home and their whole life revolves around a diet. What can a hostess serve to guests who might be on conflicting diets? Take your focus off the content of foods. Diet should not rule your life.

With all natural foods, you won't have to read labels and be obsessive about a diet. You can concentrate on the sociability of meals. Many diets in magazines and other books are too low in fiber. It's easy to drink a glass of juice instead of eating whole fruit, but you're missing nutrients. As quoted earlier, juice is to fruit as white flour is to whole-grain. With more vegetables and whole fruit in your diet and smaller amounts of meat, you wouldn't have the two symptoms that bother a lot of people on highly refined Western diets — constipation and heart burn. Your digestive system will work naturally and you won't need either over-the-counter pills or expensive prescriptions.

I think it's better to eat broad categories of food, not try to go

along with any specific diet

My personal food choices, modified over the years, might give you some ideas. They might help you change your habits and still fit your schedule. Accept some and adapt others. Don't be rigid.

Breakfasts

My breakfast for years has been one or two kinds of fruit, cut up with added cottage cheese or yogurt, topped with wheat germ, brewers' yeast and chopped nuts or sunflower seeds and a little lecithin. It's much more nutritious than cereal and milk and won't give you gas if you're lactose-intolerant. If I have eggs or waffles for breakfast, I have the fruit, nut, and dairy mixture for lunch.

I'm careful not to brown my omelets after reading that the cholesterol or proteins in the egg yolk might be changed with high heat. I cook sliced mushrooms in butter and add two eggs fork-beaten with water. The egg mixture is cooked lightly until barely set. Lately, I have found another way to incorporate vegetables into breakfast. I cut up part of an onion, chop some ginger and start them cooking in a small amount of water. I then add zucchini, bok choy or bell peppers. While I'm toasting thin slices of whole-grain bread I poach a couple of eggs with the vegetables. Sometimes I sprinkle Parmesan cheese on the toast. Sometimes I add frozen berries to applesauce and heat it in the microwave to spread on the toast.

You don't need a sweet spread. Artificial sweeteners perpetuate a craving for sweets and blunt your taste buds so you need more sweet foods more often. You can gradually get rid of a sweet tooth. First, try cranberry sauce instead of jam. Later, make your own cranberry sauce with half the sugar or use a couple tablespoons of honey instead. Try unsweetened applesauce with added cinnamon. After awhile your favorite of the four major tastes will be "sour" not "sweet".

Some days I thaw a frozen waffle and top it with berries or a mashed ripe banana. I make and freeze my own waffles every few weeks: start with two eggs beaten with 1/3 cup of olive oil. I don't measure ingredients except for one teaspoon of baking powder to each of three cups of flour. I alternate adding flour and enough buttermilk to thin the mixture. I then add a cup of whole-grain cereal (cooked in the microwave while I'm mixing other ingredients). Last I add about a tablespoon of molasses plus ½ teaspoon of baking soda to react with the acidic molasses and buttermilk. I often add brewer's yeast for its protein, vitamins and minerals.

Lunch & Dinner

Vegetables are the main part of my lunch or dinner. Two cups of salad ingredients a day are augmented with two or more large servings of cooked vegetables. Broccoli is a favorite, but I eat others in season. Lunch is sometimes a sardine salad. Some days I have white Irish cheddar cheese on whole wheat toast topped with spinach leaves or lettuce. When I make carrot juice, I save some of the high-fiber pulp. I add it to the one-third cup of lentils with chopped onions I sometimes cook for lunch. Lentils don't require soaking like beans. Split peas need to soak less than half an hour.

I always have a good quality, high-protein food for dinner. I sometimes make a stir fry, browning slices of tofu, along with sliced ginger, in olive oil. To this I add vegetables and sometimes a few frozen shrimp. I eat Alaskan salmon two or three times a week. I buy it frozen, and cut it into four-ounce pieces using a cleaver that I pound on with a hammer. I braise it in olive oil or else put it on top of sliced cooked yams in the microwave.

Selected meats

I no longer eat beef, pork or chicken since these are probably produced in factory farms. About once a week, I have four to six ounces of lamb. If I could get lamb livers, hearts and kidneys, they would be healthier than those from larger animals. Once a month, I eat chicken livers, braised in olive oil with onions and ginger and served over brown rice and chopped celery. Years ago, I could buy sweet breads (thymus gland) from an Asian grocer.

Combined with chicken livers, they made a tasty nutritious dish, high in protein, vitamins, iron and RNA.

I would like to buy organic chicken if I could get it without the breast. I think any white meat is stringy and tasteless. It seems that most diet recipes in magazines and books now imply that the only healthy meat is boneless, skinless, chicken breast. In my opinion, chicken breast is to the whole chicken as white flour is to the whole-grain. Chicken fat and skin from organic birds is healthy. Look at the liquid that comes off when you roast a chicken. When it cools, you can see that two-thirds of it is gelatin, not fat. If it's an organic chicken, that partially saturated fat is good for you.

Snacks

For a special snack, I toast whole-grain bread, spread it with cream cheese or peanut butter and add a few shavings of dark chocolate. I get the goodness of chocolate with very little sugar.

I have green tea and several herbal teas in the cupboard but rarely use them. After menopause I got muscle cramps in my legs, often if I had too much coffee. This was relieved by taking calcium. When I went on foreign trips I allowed three 500 mg. tablets per day. During an Earth Watch trip in Australia studying insects in the rain forest, I got muscle cramps every night and had to take extra calcium. I almost used up my quota. Since my final week would be scuba diving at a remote island in Fiji, I was worried about cramps, but didn't get any there. Later I decided the sulfites in the white wine we drank in Australia, while discussing the research in the evening, might have depleted my calcium. In Fiji, I drank beer, my usual beverage in a foreign country. The water is boiled to make beer and it's more healthful than soda pop.

A purist would say to protect body calcium by not drinking either coffee or alcohol. Why give up either coffee or wine? For years now I mix coffee 50:50 with a roasted grain beverage. I drink a hearty red wine diluted with water or ice. It's a middle way that works for me.

Many dieters fail because they always feel hungry

With enough fiber and good quality fat, as well as some protein with every snack or meal, you can feel satisfied for hours. You keep the right balance between glucagon and insulin. As long as you eat natural foods 95% of the time you can get healthy and stay healthy.

Remember the Golden Mean:
a balance of fat, protein & carbohydrate.

Daily Food Worksheet

Write Down the number of servings daily.

Day	Cooked Veggies	Salads	Whole Fruit	Hard Cheese	Raw Nuts
1.					
2.					
3.					
4.					
5.					
6.					
7.					
8.					
9.					
10.					
11.					
12.					
13.					
14.					
15.					
16.					
17.					
18.					
19.					
20.					
21.					

Selected Bibliography

Books:

Arvigo, Rosita and Epstein, Nadine; *Rainforest Home Remedies* (New York, Harper Collins, 2001)

Arnot, Robert; *Dr. Bob Arnot's Revolutionary Weight Control Program* (New York, Little Brown and Co., 1997)

Arnot, Robert; *Breast Cancer Prevention Diet* (New York, Warner Books, 1998)

Atkins, Robert C.; *Dr. Atkins' Age-Defying Diet* (New York, St. Martin's Press, 2001)

Austin, Denise; *Pilates for Every Body* (Rodale Press, 2002)

Bailey, Covert; *The New Fit or Fat* (Boston, Houghton Mifflin Co., 1991)

Benjamin, Samuel; *Smart Choices, Alternative Medicine* (Iowa, Better Homes and Gardens, 1999)

Berkson, Lindsey; *Hormone Deception* (Contemporary Books, 2000)

Bonner, Joseph and Harris, William; *Healthy Aging* (Claremont, Calif., Hunter House Inc., 1998)

Bragg, Paul and Bragg, Patricia; *Gourmet Health Recipes* (Santa Barbara, Calif., Health Science, 1985)

Carper, Jean; *Stop Aging Now* (New York, Harper Collins Publishers, 1995)

Chang, Henry, K.; *Weight Lost Forever* (Fair Oaks, Calif., Long Bow Publishing, 2003)

Chopra, Deepak and Simon, David; *Grow Younger Live Longer* (New York, Harmony Books, 2001)

Clower, Will; *The Fat Fallacy: French Diet Secrets to Permanent Weight Loss* (New York, 3 Rivers Press, of Random House, 2003)

Diamond, Harvey and Diamond, Marilyn; *Fit For Life II: Living Health* (New York, Warner Books, 1987)

Dobelis, Inge, et al.; *Magic and Medicine of Plants* (Pleasantville, New York, Reader's Digest Assoc., 1986)

Duke, James A.; *Handbook of Medicinal Herbs* (Boca Raton Florida, CRC Press, 2001)

Eades, Michael R. and Eades, Mary Dan; *Protein Power* (New York, Bantam Books, 1996)

Eades, Michael R. and Eades, Mary Dan; *The Protein Power Lifeplan* (New York, Warner Books, 2000)

Enig, Mary G.; *Know Your Fats: The Complete Primer on Fats and Cholesterol*

(Maryland, Bethesda Press, 2000)

Feingold, Ben and Feingold, Helene; *The Feingold Cookbook for Hyperactive Children* (New York, Random House, 1979.

Francina, Suza; *New Yoga for People Over 50* (Deerfield Beach Florida, Health Communications, 1997)

Garber, Stephen and Garber, Marianne Daniels; *Beyond Ritalin* (New York, Villard, 1996)

Gittleman, Anne Louise; *The Fat Flush Plan* (New York, McGraw Hill, 2002)

Haas, Elson; *The False Fat Diet* (New York, Ballantine Books, 2000)

Haas, Robert; *Eat to Win* (New York, Harmony Books, 2000)

Harte, John; *Toxics A to Z* (Berkeley, Calif., University of California Press, 1992)

Hausman, Patricia and Judith Benn Hurley; *Healing Foods* (Emmaus, Penn. Rodale Press, 1989)

Heller, Rachael, and Heller, Richard, *The Carbohydrate Addict's Diet* (New York, Signet, 1991)

Hockensmith, Gloria; *The Goat Doctor of the Sierras: A Healer of People* (USA, Gloriart Publishing, 2001)

Joklik, W., Willett, H. and Amos, D.B., eds.; *Zinsser Microbiology* (New York, Appleton-Century-Crofts/ Prentiss Hall, 1980)

Krimisky, Sheldon; *Hormonal Chaos: The Scientific and Social Origins of the Environmental Endocrine Hypothesis* (Baltimore, Johns Hopkins Press, 2000)

Kowalski, Robert E.; *The 8-Week Cholesterol Cure* (New York, Harper Collins, 1989)

Lesser, Michael, M.D.; *The Brain Chemistry Diet: The Personalized Prescription for Balancing Mood, Relieving Stress and Conquering Depression* (New York, G.P. Putnam and Sons, 2002)

Lipscitz, David; *Breaking the Rules of Aging* (Washington, D.C., Lifeline Press, Regnery Publishers, 2002)

Mein, Carolyn; *Different Bodies Different Diets* (New York, Regan Books, Harper Collins, 2001)

Millspaugh, Charles F.; *American Medicinal Plants* (New York, Dover Publications, Inc., 1974)

Northrup, Christiane; *Women's Bodies, Women's Wisdom* (New York, Bantam Books, 1998)

Null, Gary; *The Complete Guide to Health and Nutrition* (New York, Dell Publishing, 1978)

Null, Gary; *Gary Null's Ultimate Anti-Aging Program* (New York, Kensington Books, 1999)

Ornish, Dean; *Dr. Dean Ornish Program for Reversing Heart Disease* (New York, Random House, 1996)

Ornish, Dean; *Love and Survival* (New York, Harper Collins, 1998)

Packer, Lester; *The Antioxidant Miracle* (New York, Wiley, 1999)

Pelletier, Kenneth; *The Best Alternative Medicine* (New York, Fireside/Simon and Schuster, 2002)

Pfeiffer, Carl; *Mental and Elemental Nutrients* (New Canaan, Conn., Keats Publishers, 1975)

Pitchford, Paul; *Healing with Whole Foods* (Berkeley, North Atlantic Books, 1993)

Pritikin, Robert; *Pritikin Weight Loss Breakthrough* (New York, Penguin, a Dutton Book, 1998)

Ravnskov, Uffe; *The Cholesterol Myths* (Washington, D.C., New Trends Publishing, 2000)

Regelson, William and Colman, Carol; *The Superhormone Promise: Nature's Antidote to Aging* (New York, Simon and Schuster, 1996)

Reiter, Russel and Robinson, Jo; *Melatonin…Combat Aging, Boost Immune System, Reduce Risk of Cancer and Heart Disease, Get a Better Night's Sleep* (New York, Bantam, 1996)

Rivas, Paul; *Turn Off the Hunger Switch*: *Reset Your Brain to Change Your Weight* (New York, Hall Prentice Press, 2002)

Roberts, Arthur, O'Brien, Mary and Subak-Sharpe, Genell; *Nutraceuticals, Encyclopedia of Supplements, Herbs, Vitamins and Healing Foods* (New York, Perigree/Penguin Putnam, 2001)

Roizen, Michael; *Real Age: Are You as Young as You Can Be?* (New York, Harper Collins, 1999)

Rosenfeld, Isadore; *Dr. Rosenfeld's Guide to Alternative Medicine* (New York, Random House, 1996)

Rosenfeld, Isadore; *Live Now Age Later* (New York, Warner Books, 1999)

Rowe, John and Kahn, Robert; *Successful Aging* (New York, Pantheon Books, 1998)

Ross, Julia; *The Diet Cure: The 8-step Program to Rebalance Body Chemistry and End Food Cravings, Weight Problems and Mood Swings — Now* (New York, Penguin Books, 2000)

Schwarzbein, Diana; *The Schwarzbein Principle: The Truth About Weight Loss, Health and Aging* (Santa Barbara, Calif., Health Communications Inc., 1999)

Sears, Barry with Bill Lawren; *Enter the Zone*: *a Dietary Roadmap to Lose Weight Permanently…*(New York, Harper Collins, 1995)

Sears, Barry; *The Anti-Aging Zone* (New York, Regan/Harper Collins, 1999)

Shames, Richard L. and Shames, Karilee H.; *Thyroid Power: Ten Steps to Total Health,* (New York, Quill, Harper Collins, 2002)

Sheats, Cliff; *Lean Bodies Total Fitness* (Arlington, Texas, Summit Publishing Group, 1995)

Siegal, Sanford; *Dr. Seigal's Natural Fiber Permanent Weight Loss Diet* (New York, Dial Press, 1975)

Siegel, Bernie ; *Balanced Healing, combining modern medicine with safe, effective alternative therapies (Harbor Press, 2004)*

Smith, Timothy; *Renewal: The Anti-Aging Revolution* (Emmaus, Penn., Rodale Press, 1998)

Snyderman, Nancy; *Dr. Nancy Snyderman's Guide to Good Health* (New York, William Morrow Co., 1996)

Spiller, Gene A., editor; *Nutritional Pharmacology* (New York, A.R. Liss, 1981)

Streitwieser, Andrew and Heathcock, Clayton; *Organic Chemistry* (New York, MacMillan Publishing Co., 1981)

Victoroff, Jeff, M.D.; *Saving Your Brain* (New York, Bantam Books, 2002)

Weil, Andrew; *Eating Well for Optimum Health* (New York, Alfred A. Knopf, 2000)

Wesselman, Hank; *The Journey to the Sacred Garden* (Carlsbad, CA., Hay House Inc., 2003)

Yudkin, J.; *Sweet and Dangerous* (New York, Van Rees Press, 1972)

Zubay, Geoffrey, et al., eds.; *Biochemistry* (Reading, Mass., Addison Wesley Publishing Co., 1983)

Articles:

[Note the following abbreviations that have widespread use or acceptance are used in references: AARP is American Association of Retired Persons.
JAMA is the Journal of the American Medical Association]

Bashin, Bryan Jay; "The Freshness Illusion…Frozen Food and Serious Questions about Supermarket Produce," Harrowsmith. Jan/Feb 1987, p. 41-48.

Blair, Steven; "Physical Fitness and All Cause Mortality," JAMA 1995, 273:14:1093-9.

Bouic, Patrick and Lamprecht, Johan; "Plant Sterols and Sterolins: A Review of their Immune-Modulating Properties," Alternative Medicine Review, 1999, 4(3):170-177.

Brinton, E. and Breslow, Jan; "A low-fat diet decreases high density lipoprotein (HDL) cholesterol levels by decreasing HDL Apolipoprotein transport rates," Journal of Clinical Investigation 1990, 85:144-151.

Castelli, William; "The triglyceride issue: A View from Framingham," American Heart Journal, 1986:112:2:432-437.

Castelli, William; "Concerning the Possibility of a Nut," Archives of Internal Medicine, July, 1992, 152(7):1371-2.

Choe, M. and Yu, B.P; "Lipid peroxidation contributes to age-related membrane rigidity," Free Radical Biology and Medicine, 1995, 18:6:977-84.

Corr, L.A. and Oliver, M.F.; "The low fat, low cholesterol diet is ineffective," European Heart Journal, 1997, 18:18-32.

Cullen, P.; "Evidence that triglycerides are an independent coronary heart disease risk factor," American Journal Cardiology, 2000, 86:9:943-9.

Dyall, Donald; "Supplements are Safe- Do the Math" Letter to the Editor Health Freedom News, July-Sept., 2003.

Ellison, L.F. and Morrison, H.; "Low serum cholesterol concentration and the risk of suicide," Epidemiology, March, 2001, 12 (2):168-72.

Fraser, Gary, et al.; "Possible Protection of Nut Consumption on the Risk of Coronary Heart Disease," Archives of Internal Medicine, 1992, 152:1416-1424.

Fuhrman-Bianca, O. J., et al.; "Increased Uptake of LDL by Oxidized Macrophages is the Result of an Initial enhanced LDL Receptor Activity and the Progressive Oxidation of LDL", Free Radical Biology and Medicine, 1997, 23:1:34-46.

Gaziano, J.M., et al.; "Fasting Triglycerides, High-Density Lipoprotein, and Risk of Myocardial Infarction," Circulation, 1997, 96:2520-24.

Gillman, M.W, Cupples, L.W., Millen, B.E., Ellison, R.C. and Wolf, P.A.; "Inverse association of dietary fat with development of ischemic stroke in men," JAMA, 1997:278:24: 2145-50.

Gwinup, G.; "Effect of Exercise Alone on the Weight of Obese Women," Archives of Internal Medicine 1975, 135:676-80.

Harjai, K.J.; "Potential new cardiovascular risk factors: Left ventricular hypertrophy, homocysteine, lipoprotein (a), triglycerides, oxidative stress and fibrinogen," Annals of Internal Medicine, 1999 131:376-86.

Hayek, T.I., et al.; "Dietary fat increases high density lipoprotein (HDL) levels both by increasing the transport rates and decreasing the fractional catabolic rates of HDL cholesterol ester and apolipoprotein (apo A-1)," Journal of Clinical Investigation, 1993, 91:1667-1671.

Horrobin, D.; "The Importance of Gamma-Linolenic Acid and Prostaglandin E 1 in Human Nutrition and Medicine," Journal of Holistic Medicine, 1981, 3:118-139.

Hu, Frank B., et al.; "Risk of Coronary Heart Disease in Women: Harvard Nurses Study," New England Journal of Medicine, 1995, 337:1491-99.

Hu, Frank B., et al.; "A prospective study of egg consumption and risk of cardiovascular disease in men and women," JAMA, 1999, 281:15:1387-94.

Kritchevsky D.; "History of recommendations to the public about dietary fat," Journal of Nutrition 1998, 128:449S–452S.

Leon, A., et al.; "Effects of a Vigorous Walking Program on Body Composition and Metabolism of Obese Young Men," Journal of Clinical Nutrition, 1979, 32:1776-87.

Libby, P.; "Atherosclerosis, the New View," Scientific American, May, 2002, 47-55.

Liu, Simin, Willet, W.C., et al.; "A prospective study of dietary glycemic load, carbohydrate intake and risk of coronary heart disease in U.S. women," American Journal of Clinical Nutrition, 2000, 71:1455-61.

Montgomery, Anne; "America's Pesticide Permeated Food," Nutrition Action Health Newsletter, June, 1987, pp. 1-4.

Moroney, J.T., et al.; "Low-density lipoprotein cholesterol and the risk of dementia with stroke," JAMA ,1999, 282:254-260.

Morrow, D.A. and Ricker, P.M.; "C-Reactive Protein, a diagnostic marker of inflammation," Circulation Research, 2001, 89:763.

Pollan, Michael; "The (Agri)cultural Contradictions of Obesity," New York Times, Oct.12, 2003.

Rapaport, Lisa; "CalPERS study on managing disease," The Sacramento Bee, June 15, 2003

Ravnskov, U.; "The Questionable Role of Saturated and Polyunsaturated Fatty Acids in Cardiovascular Disease," Journal of Clinical Epidemiology, 1998, 51:6:443-60.

Robinson, K., Mayer, E. and Jacobsen, D.W.; "Homocysteine and coronary artery disease," Cleveland Clinic Journal of Medicine, 1994, 61:438-50.

Sapolsky, R.M.; "Why stress is bad for your brain," Science 1996, 273:749-50.

Sherman, B.B.; "Estrogen and cognitive functioning in women," Proceedings of Society of Biology and Medicine, 1998, 217:17-22.

Sugarman, Carole; "Facing the Issue of Pesticide Residues," Washington Post, June 3, 1987.

Sloop, G.D.; "A critical analysis of the role of cholesterol in atherogenesis," Atherosclerosis, 1999, 142:265-268.

Velez-Carrasco, W., et al.; "Dietary restriction of saturated fat and cholesterol decreases HDL ApoA-1 secretion," Arteriosclerosis, Thrombo-Vascular Biology, April 19, 1999, 4:918-24.

Willett, W.C., et al.; "Relation of meat, fat and fiber to the risk of colon cancer in a prospective study among women," New England Journal of Medicine, 1990, 323:24:1664-1665.

Willett, W.C., et al.; "Dietary fat and fiber in relation to risk of breast cancer," JAMA, 1992, 268:15:2037.

Yaffe, K., et. al.; "Estrogen therapy in post-menopausal women: effect on cognitive function and dementia," JAMA, 1996, 279:698-695.

Young, B., Gleeson, M. and Cripps, A."C-reactive protein: A critical review," Pathology, 1991, 23:118-124.

Other Sources:

AARP Bulletin ; "The Nursing Squeeze", May, 2003.

AARP Bulletin; "Overmedicating America", November, 2003.

AARP Bulletin; "The Pharmacist Who Says No to Drugs", September, 2004

Block, Mary Ann, D.O.; "The overuse of Ritalin," on Montel Williams, NBC, April 15, 2003.

Consumer's Guidebook by Center for Study of Responsive Law; *Eating Clean Overcoming Food Hazards*. Order from Eating Clean, P.O. Box 19367, Washington, D.C., 2003

Fallest-Strobl, Patricia, et. al.; "Homocysteine: A New Risk Factor for Atherosclerosis,"
University of Wisconsin, Madison, Medical School,
www.aafp.org/afp/971015ap/fallest.html 2002.

Hunt, Janeen; "A Review of Diet, Fat and Cholesterol Research: 25 Points,"
j_hunt@immutopicsintl.com , 2002.

Kenney, James J.; "Fructose Raises Cholesterol," excerpted from Diet and Cardiovascular Disease, *www.foodandhealth.com/fructose.shtml,* 2002.

Oldways Preservation and Exchange Trust, 266 Beacon Street, Boston, MA 02116,
www.oldways.org

Reichman, Judith; " Smoking increases risk of cardiac death by 3,000 percent," NBC Jan. 7, 2002.

South, James; "Weight Loss the Anti-Aging Way," Nov. 29, 2001, pp. 1-19,
www.smart-drugs.net/ias-weightloss.html

Wesselman, Hank, A workshop on shamanic drumming at the Learning Exchange, Sacramento, Feb. 14-16, 2003. www.sharedwisdom.com

Sources For Buying Healthy Foods:

Niman Ranch; 1025 E. 12th St., Oakland, CA 94606. Phone 866.808.0340, fax: 510.808.0339. Niman Ranch sells quality, organic meats raised humanely. It coordinates with many small family farms, inspecting their land and methods. It processes the beef, pork and lamb from these farms. It sells nationally to consumers as well as restaurants and retailers (such as Trader Joes) *www.nimanranch.com*

Organic Valley Family of Farms; CROPP Cooperative, One Organic Way, LaFarge, WI 54639. Phone: 888.444.6455, fax: 608.625.3025. This cooperative consists of 600 farmers nationwide who practice sustainable agriculture. They produce organic milk, juice, eggs, meat and produce. (Call to find out where to buy their products).

Weight, Measurement & Activity Worksheet

Initial Weight: *Measurement of Abdomen:*
Measurement of Chest: *Measurement of Hips:*

Day	Exercise type	Minutes or Hours
1.		
2.		
3.		
4.		
5.		
6.		
7.		
8.		
9.		
10.		
11.		
12.		
13.		
14.		
15.		
16.		
17.		
18.		
19.		
20.		
21.		

Index

Golden Green Press Quick Order Form

Phone orders: 916-966-3453

email orders or questions: goldengreen@calweb .com.

Postal orders: Golden Green Press
PO Box 1087
Fair Oaks CA 95628-1087

Send To:

Name _____

Address _____

_____

City _____ State _____ Zip _____

Telephone _____ Fax: _____

Email address _____

Notes: _____

_____

Send _____ copies of ***Don't Get Thin Get Healthy*** @ $18.95 each

Total for books $_____

Sales Tax: Add 7.75% for books shipped to California $_____

Postage: $4.^{00} for one book, $2.^{00} each for additional books $_____

(U.S. only. International orders, call or e-mail)

TOTAL ORDER $_____

Enclose payment (check or money order) made out to "Golden Green Press"
Prices subject to change without notice. Allow 2-3 weeks for delivery.
Wholesale orders: call the office, 9 am - 5pm PST